Student Workbook to Accompany

Contemporary Medical Office Procedures

Third Edition

Doris D. Humphrey, Ph.D.

President, Career Solutions Training Group

THOMSON

DELMAR LEARNING™

Australia Canada Mexico Singapore Spain United Kingdom United States

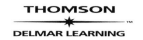

THOMSON

DELMAR LEARNING

Student Workbook to Accompany Contemporary Medical Office Procedures, Third Edition
by Doris D. Humphrey, PhD

Vice President, Health Care SBU:
William Brottmiller

Editorial Director:
Cathy L. Esperti

Acquisitions Editor:
Rhonda Dearborn

Editorial Assistant:
Natalie Wager

Developmental Editor:
Mary Ellen Cox

Marketing Director:
Jennifer McAvey

Channel Manager:
Lisa Osgood

Marketing Coordinator:
Mona Caron

Technology Specialist:
Victoria Moore

Production Coordinator:
Jessica Peterson

Project Editor:
Bryan Viggiani

Art and Design Coordinator:
Connie Lundberg-Watkins

NOTICE TO THE READER

Table of Contents

Preface

As the physician's job has become more complex under managed care, the medical assistant's responsibilities have broadened. Medical assistants are expected to apply knowledge in many areas, ranging from understanding the highly legislated managed care community to interacting with patients and coordinating the daily schedule, to using sophisticated technology for communication and record keeping, to demonstrating in-depth critical thinking and problem-solving skills. The dynamic, often rushed, atmosphere of a medical setting requires each medical assistant to demonstrate an excellent attitude—one that translates into cooperation, acceptance of responsibility, and the desire to continue learning.

This *Student Workbook to Accompany Contemporary Medical Office Procedures,* Third Edition, was written to help the learner review concepts presented in the textbook and to assist students in gaining the knowledge and skills needed to be successful. It encourages the application of medical office assisting knowledge in a variety of learning situations. It may be used with the *Contemporary Medical Office Procedures* textbook or as a text-workbook for short segments of learning or individualized study. This student workbook can be incorporated into many classes with varying time schedules.

Suggestions for Using the Student Workbook

Each chapter of the workbook extends the material contained in the matching chapters of the textbook. Look for these components:

- Key Vocabulary Terms test the students' knowledge of the chapter vocabulary.

- Chapter Review questions assess the students' understanding of the chapter content.

- Critical Thinking Scenarios challenge the students to assume the role of a medical office assistant and make decisions.

- "Day-in-the-Life" Simulations require students to perform real-life tasks that they might encounter in a medical practice.

- The workbook is correlated to Delmar's Medical Assisting CD-ROM. Most chapters of the workbook direct students to the CD-ROM to complete an activity.

- The instructor's manual for *Contemporary Medical Office Procedures,* Third Edition, includes a special section devoted to the workbook. In this section, you will find solutions to all chapter activities and recommended answers to the Day-in-the-Life simulations.

Name: _____ Date: _____

PART I   Today's Medical Environment

CHAPTER 1
The Medical Environment

Chapter Outline

Key Vocabulary Terms

Match each word or term with its correct meaning.

_____ 1. On call   a. concentration on specific body systems

_____ 2. CDC   b. full bill paid each time a patient visits the physician

_____ 3. Third-party reimbursement   c. physicians and hospitals compete for patients

_____ 4. Fee-for-service   d. three years of specialty training

_____ 5. Managed competition   e. basic medical word plus prefix or suffix

_____ 6. Medical specialties   f. availability on an as-needed basis

_____ 7. Residency   g. someone other than the patient pays

_____ 8. Root medical word   h. Atlanta research center

Chapter Review

1. Why are health care costs rising in the United States?

_____

_____

_____

_____

2. How have high costs of medical care changed the physician's work?

_____

_____

_____

_____

3. How have the high costs of medical care affected the medical assistant's work?

_____

_____

_____

_____

4. How do the rising costs of medical malpractice insurance affect society?

_____

_____

_____

_____

5. What factors are contributing to the increase in jobs available for medical assistants?

_____

_____

_____

_____

6. Why is documentation of medical records more important today than ever before?

_____

_____

_____

_____

7. Why are group practices becoming more common among doctors?

_____

_____

_____

_____

8. In what ways has the Centers for Medicare & Medicaid Services affected medical assistants?

_____

_____

_____

_____

9. What importance has the Health Insurance Portability Act had on health care reform?

_____

_____

_____

_____

10. Computers are used in medicine for many administrative and diagnostic purposes. For each of the following, write an *A* to identify the purpose as *Administrative* and a *D* to identify the purpose as *Diagnostic*.

_____ Analyze and refine patient data from laboratory tests

_____ Maintain a record of a patient's health

_____ Suggest an illness after test results are entered

_____ Cross-check drugs

_____ Show magnetic resonance imaging scans

_____ Store and access a physician's instructions to nurses

_____ Maintain a database of correct dosages based on patient weight

_____ Send a picture of a patient's heart from a remote location to a large hospital

_____ Analyze and interpret information about a diseased body part

Critical Thinking Scenarios

1. Wicha Rafer soon will be graduating from a two-year medical assisting program. Recently, she had the following conversation with a friend. Assume you are the friend. What advice will you give Wicha?

   "I just can't decide whether to work in a solo practice or a group practice. The idea of working in a big practice with several doctors is exciting, but it's also appealing to think that in a solo practice I would work closely with one doctor. I don't think I have any other choices though. What's your advice?"

   _____

   _____

   _____

   _____

   _____

   _____

2. After sending out resumes for six weeks, your neighbor, Joel Reddy, has been called to interview for a medical assistant position at two practices. One practice contracts with an EPO, and the other is part of an HMO that offers a Point-of-Service Plan. Joel calls you in a panic the night before the first interview and says, "I still get confused about what all these acronyms mean. Tell me again what the difference is between an EPO and a POS Plan."

_____

_____

_____

_____

3. During your internship rotation as a medical assistant, you had an opportunity to work in three different specialties or subspecialties: a dermatology practice, a family practice, and an emergency medicine practice. A student who is just entering the medical assisting program asks you to describe what each practice does and the type of patients it sees. What will you tell her?

_____

_____

_____

_____

_____

4. As program director for your local AAMA chapter, you have invited a panel of dental specialists to discuss job opportunities in their field. To start the program, you will introduce the dentists, then give a short summary of the dental specialties of the American Dental Association. You have two minutes for your part of the program.

_____

_____

_____

5. The young endocrinologist for whom you work is thinking about developing a research project using his patients as subjects. He is interested in many different disorders and illnesses, so he is open to researching in a variety of areas. He believes that he can secure funding for the research from either the Centers for Disease Control and Prevention or the National Institutes of Health. Because of his busy schedule, he asks you to research the Internet for available grants, then to summarize for him the work these two leading institutions are doing. Use the following Web sites for your research: http://www.cdc.gov and http://www.nih.gov.

_____

_____

_____

6. You have been invited back to the school where you received your medical assisting training to speak to a class of entering medical assistants. The new students are very focused. Within weeks of the start of school, many already have decided what area of medicine interests them most as a field of work; however, some have not yet connected their interests with the body systems. Tell Clarissa, Alan, Maria, Pia, Juan, Anna, Ling, and Sean the body system that relates most closely to their interests.

_____ Clarissa is a former gymnast. She would like to combine her interest in medicine with body movement.

_____ As a child, Alan's bloody cuts and scrapes were fascinating because they usually healed without help from a doctor. When he was older, he routinely volunteered to donate blood and volunteered at the Red Cross. The role of blood to body functioning intrigues him.

_____ Maria loves babies, and stories about difficult pregnancies, premature births, problem deliveries, and infertility capture her interest.

_____ Pia is a brain; everyone says so. Therefore, it is no surprise that she is interested in how the brain tells the body what to do and how to do it.

_____ Juan's mom was sick until she was diagnosed with hyperthyroidism and swallowed radioactive iodine to eliminate her thyroid gland. Since then, Juan has been amazed at her progress. He would like to work in a field that helps him learn more about this and similar illnesses.

_____ Anna's animals were easy to identify in her neighborhood as she was growing up, for their legs were usually in a cast. At one point, she adopted a three-legged pug who ended up with a peg leg of her design. It is a foregone conclusion that she wants to work with broken bones.

_____ After Ling's grandma died of lung cancer and his uncle was sick for years with emphysema, there was never a question that he would work with a doctor who treats these illnesses.

_____ Sean was an EMT in high school and saw many burn victims whose lost large portions of their skin in fires. He has witnessed the terrible suffering and the miraculous healing that can occur when the skin is involved, and he is determined to learn more.

circulatory system	the heart, blood vessels, blood, and lymphatic system
digestive system	organs and glands associated with ingestion and digestion of food
endocrine system	glands that regulate body functions, including the adrenal, pituitary, thyroid, and sex glands
integumentary system	nails, hair, skin and related appendages
muscular system	more than 600 muscles that contract and pull tissue to create body movement
nervous system	brain, spinal cord, and others that regulate and coordinate the activities of all the other systems
respiratory system	organs that allow breathing
reproductive system	organs that enable men and women to have children
skeletal system	bones that support and protect the body
urinary system	filters wastes from the blood and flushes them from the body through urine

Simulations Introduction

The simulations you are about to begin represent the work you will perform during your first fifteen days at Graupera and Marks—one simulation for each day. After completing all fifteen simulations, one referenced to each chapter of the textbook, you will have experienced most of the activities typically performed by a medical assistant in any private practice. Save all the Action Papers in each simulation because you will need them later.

Simulation Scenario

Your First Job

Congratulations! You have just been hired by Dr. Judith Marks and Dr. Ramon Graupera, specialists in internal medicine and cardiology at Marks and Graupera, P.C., 2201 Locust Street, Philadelphia, PA 19101. Telephone: 215-283-8372; fax: 215-283-2938; e-mail: MG@MarksandGraupera.com. You are on your way to an exciting career in Philadelphia, Pennsylvania.

Medical assisting positions with Dr. Marks, the senior physician and cardiologist, and Dr. Graupera, the managing physician and internal medical specialist, are coveted because the doctors expect a great deal from their staff and reward them with interesting challenges and excellent pay. They provide all new medical assistants with three weeks of intensive training that is thorough, challenging, and enjoyable. Working with these well-respected physicians is prestigious and forms the foundation for a rewarding career.

You will work with other staff members. Suzanne Romez, a physician's assistant, and Luke Streeter, a clinical medical assistant, report to Dr. Marks. Lydia Makay, CMA, office manager; Tarik Loper, clinical administrative assistant; and you, report to Dr. Graupera.

Dr. Marks is a 1965 graduate of the University of Pennsylvania School of Medicine and Dr. Graupera is a 1963 graduate of Vanderbilt University School of Medicine. Dr. Marks's Social Security number is 415-55-4321 and Dr. Graupera's Social Security number is 365-55-1061.

Marks and Graupera is located in downtown Philadelphia, near Independence Hall, the Liberty Bell, and the Constitution Center. Benjamin Franklin is buried nearby and George Washington led the Battle of Valley Forge a few miles away. The Hospital of the University of Pennsylvania, Pennsylvania Children's Hospital, and Jefferson Hospital are a short walk or taxi ride away. You are lucky in many ways; you will be working for great doctors and walking on the same streets as the signers of the Declaration of Independence and will be near some of America's most prestigious medical research and treatment centers.

Good luck in your new position.

Simulation Preparation

1. Prepare fifteen file folders with labels—one file folder for each of fifteen simulations. Label each folder with the simulation number and your name (Simulation 1: First name and last name).

2. Before starting a simulation, review the chapter in the textbook that the simulation matches. For example, Chapter 1 should be reviewed before beginning Simulation 1.

Simulation Procedures

1. Organize the Action Papers for the simulation in numerical order. Keep all papers for the simulation together. Read each of the papers, including all handwritten instructions.

2. Rate the urgency of each task using the categories below:

   Rush—Tasks on which action should be taken immediately

   ASAP—Tasks on which action should be taken as soon as all Rush items are completed

   Routine—Tasks that can be carried over to another day, if necessary

3. Mark the urgency of each Action Paper in Section 1 of the Work Summary (found at the end of the chapter). To do this, list each Action Paper number (shown in the upper right corner of the Action Paper) in its correct category: Rush, ASAP, or Routine. Your instructor will use the Work Summary for evaluation purposes.

4. Complete a To Do List with a brief description of each action to be taken. You will find a blank To Do List following the Action Papers.

5. Read the Supplies Needed and the Action Options, Suggestions, and Conflicts sections that come right before the Action Papers begin. Gather the supplies you will need (many are included in your workbook, but there are some things you will need to supply, such as blank paper), then perform the tasks indicated by each Action Paper. Some tasks will include instructions, whereas the proper handling of others will be left for you to decide on. Because your time each day in the medical office is limited, and patients generate a great deal of work, use the most efficient processes and procedures to complete each task.

6. Check off each task on your To Do List as it is completed.

7. Place each Action Paper in its simulation folder. Clip to it any accompanying papers you generate.

8. Follow the same procedure with the next simulation.

9. Merge leftover work from a previous day with the next day's papers and reprioritize as needed.

Simulation 1

Supplies Needed

Reply e-mail form
Blank note form
Blank paper
To Do List
Work Summary

Action Options, Suggestions, and Conflicts

- Use the blank e-mail forms that are provided if you do not have access to e-mail, or key and print e-mail messages directly from the computer if you have access to e-mail.

- Telephone conversations are identified by an illustration of a telephone at the top of an Action Paper.

- Face-to-face conversations are identified by an illustration of people at the top of an Action Paper.

- When reference is made to a CD-ROM, use the CD-ROM that accompanies your textbook. These activities are identified by an illustration of a CD at the top of an Action Paper.

- If a form becomes too messy to use because of corrections or other reasons, obtain and copy a blank form from your instructor or use plain paper. Label the form appropriately.

Please complete the chart so you'll have a clear idea of the reporting order.
Lydia

Organization Chart

```
┌──────────────────────────────────────────────────────────────────┐
│                                                                    │
│                      _____                      │
│                           Name of Practice                         │
│                                                                    │
└──────────────────────────────────────────────────────────────────┘

┌────────────────────────────┐        ┌────────────────────────────┐
└────────────────────────────┘        └────────────────────────────┘
   Senior Physician and Specialty         Managing Physician and Specialty

                                          ┌──────────────────────────┐
                                          └──────────────────────────┘
                                                 Office Manager

┌─────────────┐  ┌─────────────┐     ┌─────────────┐  ┌─────────────┐
│             │  │             │     │             │  │             │
└─────────────┘  └─────────────┘     └─────────────┘  └─────────────┘
  Physician's       Clinical          Administrative      Clinical
   Assistant    Medical Assistant    Medical Assistant  Medical Assistant
```

Name: _____   Date: _____

Action Paper 1-2

To: Your name@MarksandGraupera.com
From: TarikLoper@MarksandGraupera.com
Subject: Lunch

Hi, you've been in meetings with Lydia all morning, so I haven't had a chance to say much more than hello. Would you like to go to lunch? I'll fill you in on some of the things you'll need to know.

I'm glad you came to work here. You'll like it. Dr. Graupera is great. So is Dr. Marks, but you won't see as much of her.

E-mail me back about lunch.

Reply To: TarikLoper@MarksandGraupera.com
From: Your name@MarksandGraupera.com
Subject: Lunch

Dr. Graupera: "I just finished a brief examination of Maryellen Reynolds, who is still in the examining room. Write Tarik a note to schedule her for a complete physical exam and an electrocardiogram, then to send her to the lab for a complete blood count, a thyroid profile, and a urinalysis. Tell him to give her written instructions of the medications: Tylenol as needed and at bedtime. By the way, use medical abbreviations in your note to Tarik. That's what he is used to seeing."

You: "All right, I will."

Action Paper 1-4

Tarik: "A few years ago we made up a glossary of the words and terms that our practice uses frequently. It has been very helpful to me, and we've recorded it on CD for new medical assistants. Here's my copy of the CD. Why don't you look at the terms and start a notebook of any definitions you aren't familiar with, in case the docs use a term you don't know."

You: "Thanks."

Action Paper 1-5

Marks and Graupera, P.C.

Note from Lydia

Sorry I had to run out on you. The accountant called, and I had to spend some time with him. How about us continuing our meeting at lunch? There's a good place nearby where we can have a sandwich and finish up the details that will help you get started. I'll be busy tomorrow so we won't have a chance to spend too much time together. Write a note on this sheet and leave it on my desk telling me what time you prefer to go. I'm flexible.

Lydia

Name: _____   Date: _____

To Do List

-
-
-
-
-
-
-
-
-
-
-
-
-
-
-
-

Name: _____

Date Started: _____ Date Completed: _____

Work Summary 1

Section 1

1. Record the numbers of the Action Papers marked "Rush." _____

2. Record the numbers of the Action Papers marked "ASAP." _____

3. Record the numbers of the Action Papers marked "Routine." _____

Section 2

4. Write the list of "To Do" items and the actions that were taken. When this section is complete, turn the Work Summary over to your instructor, who will evaluate your work and return it for your later use.

To Do   Action Taken

_____   _____

_____   _____

_____   _____

_____   _____

_____   _____

_____   _____

Section 3

5. You will receive two assessments for your work—one is based on time to complete the items and the other is based on quality of work. Your instructor will complete the Assessment portion of the Work Summary.

Points Received

Time Required   _____
            20 points   25 minutes or less
            15 points   30 minutes
            10 points   35 minutes
             5 points   40 minutes

Quality of Work   _____

                              Total Points _____

CHAPTER 2
The Medical Staff

Chapter Outline

The Medical Assistant
    Certification
    Career Opportunities
    The Multiskilled Medical Assistant
    Responsibilities of the Position
    The Role Delineation Study Analysis
    Job Titles and Job Sites
The Roles of Medical Professionals
    Physicians
    Physician Extenders
    Nurses
    Medical Technologists and Technicians
    Medical Records Personnel
Working with the Medical Professionals
    Working with the Physician and the Health Care Team
        Honesty
        Cooperation
        Assertiveness
        Dependability
        Loyalty
    Coordinating with the Hospital Staff
    Interacting with Other Outside Professionals
Chapter Activities
    Performance-Based Activities
    Expanding Your Thinking

Key Vocabulary Terms

Match each word or term with its correct meaning.

_____ 1. Ambulatory care centers	a. trained support staff for physician
_____ 2. CMA	b. Role Delineation Chart
_____ 3. CPT	c. administrative and clinical training
_____ 4. Credentialing	d. twenty-four-hour medical centers
_____ 5. Multiskilled medical assistant	e. medical assistant accrediting group
_____ 6. OMA	f. Current Procedural Terminology
_____ 7. Physician extenders	g. medical assistant organization
_____ 8. RMA	h. Certified Medical Assistant
_____ 9. AAMA	i. examination for office procedures
_____ 10. CAAHEP	j. Registered Medical Assistant
_____ 11. RDC	k. Ophthalmic Medical Assistant

Chapter Review

1. Name several specific job titles, such as receptionist, that fall under the broad category of medical assistant.

   _____

   _____

   _____

   _____

2. How does an administrative medical assistant's work differ from the work of a clinical medical assistant and a multiskilled medical assistant?

   _____

   _____

   _____

   _____

3. What is required to become a Certified Medical Assistant?

   _____

   _____

   _____

   _____

4. Name several responsibilities of an administrative medical assistant.

   _____

   _____

   _____

   _____

5. Name several responsibilities of a clinical medical assistant.

   _____

   _____

   _____

   _____

6. Why is the Role Delineation Chart important?

_____

_____

_____

_____

7. What suppport does a medical assistant provide to a physician?

_____

_____

_____

_____

8. Identify several tasks of a support nature that medical assistants perform to help other medical professionals in the office.

_____

_____

_____

_____

9. Why is the medical assistant job category growing in number of positions?

_____

_____

_____

_____

10. Why are job opportunities better for a certified medical assistant than for a noncertified medical assistant?

_____

_____

_____

_____

_____

Critical Thinking Scenarios

1. After graduating from a medical assisting program, you decide to expand your knowledge of the United States by starting your career in another city. After researching the Internet, you discover the number of medical assisting positions that are projected to be available this year in six cities. Because you are not sure whether you prefer to work in a primary care, surgical, or other specialty, you use the percentages published by the AAMA to calculate approximately how many positions might be available in each specialty in each city. Based on the information in the AAMA chart on page 21 of the textbook, calculate and list the numbers in each position in each city.

   City No. 1   219 positions total

   _____ primary care   _____ surgical   _____ other

   City No. 2   529 positions total

   _____ primary care   _____ surgical   _____ other

   City No. 3   370 positions total

   _____ primary care   _____ surgical   _____ other

   City No. 4   134 positions total

   _____ primary care   _____ surgical   _____ other

   City No. 5   77 positions total

   _____ primary care   _____ surgical   _____ other

   City No. 6   402 positions total

   _____ primary care   _____ surgical   _____ other

2. Tuan, Rebecca, and Judy have applied at the dermatology practice where you work as an office manager. From their descriptions, which person do you think should specialize in **administrative tasks**, which should specialize in **clinical tasks**, and which should pursue a job that involves **multiple skills**.

   _____ Tuan likes to work alone where he can concentrate on a task or a puzzling problem. Though he enjoys being around people occasionally, he often becomes tired and irritable when he is surrounded by others. Tuan is great with details, and you can trust any work he does to be complete and accurate.

   _____ Rebecca has been juggling projects as long as she can remember. She is active in many different groups and often is appointed as the group's leader because she can be depended on to follow through until a project is completed. She likes to know how to do many different things, and she works hard to be good at what she does. In fact, Rebecca gets bored if she has to concentrate on one thing for too long.

   _____ Judy puts people at ease in difficult situations. She gains their confidence and is able to help them overcome their insecurities. She is one of those people you can trust to make you feel better because her personality is warm and caring. Judy is surprised that she is known as a "people person" because her real love is science and physiology, a field that is more focused on facts and statistics.

3. Ratha starts next week as a medical assistant in the pediatric practice where you work. Several individuals with different titles work at Pediatric Partners, P.C., and Ratha wants to become as knowledgeable as possible about their responsibilities before her first day. She asks you to tell her what each staff member does. Later, she will determine in what way she will be working with each.

Dr. Romez, pediatrician

_____

_____

_____

_____

Anita, physician assistant

_____

_____

_____

_____

Gordon, medical technologist

_____

_____

_____

_____

Sung-Li, medical records technician

_____

_____

_____

_____

4. As senior medical assistant at Chairson and Lopez, P.C., you have been assigned to mentor Kathi Polenski, who came to work four weeks ago. Lately, you have made notes about Kathi's observable behaviors that concern you. Now it is time to talk to her. Kathi has strong opinions and says what she thinks. One staff member has called Kathi "pushy" and says she is uncooperative. As you have watched the situation unfold, you have come to believe that Kathi is like many new graduates who need to aggressively establish how smart they are because they think they gain respect. What will you say?

_____

_____

_____

_____

5. As a medical assistant at Devon Medical Center, you have learned that working with other staff is often a challenge. Sometimes it is hard to know the right thing to do. A conversation you had with another medical assistant this morning (shown below) is disturbing, and you are trying to decide how you should have handled it. What should you have done?

   Duana: "Dr. Bolling's schedule for tomorrow morning shows she's out until 10:00 on a personal appointment. Don't tell anyone I said this, but I think she's pregnant and trying to hide it. I saw her coming out of the OB/GYN's office on the third floor when I took the elevator yesterday. Since she's going to be late, I'm going to sneak in late, too. Cover for me, and she'll never know. I shouldn't be more than thirty minutes late."

   _____

   _____

   _____

   _____

6. Duana, identified above, guessed wrong. Dr. Bolling arrived on time this morning, as did a patient she had consulted with on the phone last night and had asked to come in early. You are busy with a patient of Dr. Janeway's and can offer minimum assistance. Dr. Bolling appears irritated and asks you why Duana is late.

   _____

   _____

   _____

   _____

7. You are attending a seminar on "Managing the Administrative Staff" after being promoted to office manager at Frazier Radiology Associates. As part of a small group discussion, you are asked to name and discuss the traits you think are most important in getting along with other staff, including the physicians.

   _____

   _____

   _____

   _____

8. Shyness is a trait you wish you could overcome. You do your job well; you are well respected and you feel comfortable with yourself most of the time. But you hate confrontation and often agree to things when you would prefer to disagree. At lunch, you are so frustrated that you complain about yourself to Elana, your friend. She says, "I know what I think, but you tell me what you can do to change."

   _____

   _____

   _____

   _____

Simulation 2

Today is your second day of work at Marks and Graupera. Review the Simulation Preparation and Procedures instructions from Simulation 1 and process today's papers in the same manner.

Supplies Needed

Role Delineation Chart
Blank paper
Notepaper
To Do List
Work Summary

Action Options, Suggestions, and Conflicts

Several things you need to think about as you make decisions today are listed below.

- At lunch today, you are planning to return a pair of pants that are too large.
- Lydia has scheduled you to spend the afternoon getting up-to-date on the computer system. She has asked you to plan to work with another employee from 1:00 to 5:00, the normal end of the day. Tonight you are meeting a friend at the gym at 5:30 to work out.

Action Paper 2-1

Marks and Graupera, P.C.

Note from Dr. Marks

Sorry I was out of the office for your first day of work. We are pleased you have joined us. You had excellent references, and we're expecting great things from you. I would like to spend some time with you this afternoon. I am available at 1:30, 4:30, and 5:45. Please return this note telling me your preference.

Name: _____   Date: _____

Action Paper 2-2

To: Your name@MarksandGraupera.com
From: TarikLoper@MarksandGraupera.com
Subject: Lunch

Do you still have my CD of the practice's glossary? Getting familiar with a few more terms with help you since we use them a lot. Why don't you add these to the notebook we talked about?

professional courtesy
nonverbal behavior
pharmaceutical representative
health maintenance organization
employee handbook

professional
medical assistant
oral communication skills
employee
partnership

Marks and Graupera, P.C.

Note from Tarik

Since Lydia preempted me yesterday at lunch, let's try to go to lunch today. The office closes from 12:00 to 1:00 every day for lunch. Let me know.

T. L.

Name: _____   Date: _____

Action Paper 2-4

To: Your name@MarksandGraupera.com
From: LydiaMakay@MarksandGraupera.com
Subject: Task list

To get you off to a good start, Dr. Graupera and I would like to assign tasks that take advantage of your best skills and strengths. Will you please rate your skill level in each area on the attached chart as Basic, Above Average, or Excellent? Thanks.

Marks and Graupera Task List
Taken from the AAMA Role Delineation Chart

Administrative Procedures

_____ Perform basic clerical functions

_____ Perform basic administrative medical assisting functions

_____ Schedule, coordinate, and monitor appointments

_____ Schedule inpatient/outpatient admissions and procedures

_____ Understand and apply third-party guidelines

_____ Obtain reimbursement through accurate claims submission

_____ Monitor third-party reimbursement

_____ Understand and adhere to managed care policies and procedures

_____ *Negotiate managed care contracts

Practice Finance

_____ Perform procedural and diagnostic testing

_____ Apply bookkeeping principles

_____ Manage accounts receivable

_____ *Manage accounts payable

_____ *Process payroll

_____ *Document and maintain accounting and banking records

_____ *Document and maintain fee schedules

_____ *Manage renewals of business and professional insurance policies

_____ *Manage personnel benefits and maintain records

_____ *Perform marketing, financial, and strategic planning

*Denotes advanced skills.

Name: _____   Date: _____

Caller: Hi, it's Janie, how is the new job?

You: I like it.

Caller: Remember when we talked a few weeks ago, and I said I was thinking about pursuing CMA certification? You seemed to know a lot about certification. I can't remember everything you said. When you have a chance, will you send me an e-mail of what I have to do to become certified?

You: Sure, as soon as I get a chance.

To Do List

-
-
-
-
-
-
-
-
-
-
-
-
-
-
-
-

Name: _____

Date Started: _____ Date Completed: _____

Work Summary 2

Section 1

1. Record the numbers of the Action Papers marked "Rush." _____

2. Record the numbers of the Action Papers marked "ASAP." _____

3. Record the numbers of the Action Papers marked "Routine." _____

Section 2

4. Write the list of "To Do" items and the actions that were taken. When this section is complete, turn the Work Summary over to your instructor, who will evaluate your work and return it for your later use.

To Do   Action Taken

_____   _____

_____   _____

_____   _____

_____   _____

_____   _____

_____   _____

Section 3

5. You will receive two assessments for your work—one is based on time to complete the items and the other is based on quality of work. Your instructor will complete the Assessment portion of the Work Summary.

                                                                Points Received

Time Required   _____
                20 points   25 minutes or less
                15 points   30 minutes
                10 points   35 minutes
                 5 points   40 minutes

Quality of Work   _____

                                         Total Points _____

CHAPTER 3
Medical Ethics

Chapter Outline

Key Vocabulary Terms

Match each word or term with its correct meaning.

_____ 1. Bioethics
_____ 2. DNR
_____ 3. Durable power of attorney
_____ 4. Genetic counseling
_____ 5. Genetic engineering
_____ 6. Genetics
_____ 7. Living will
_____ 8. Medical ethics
_____ 9. Medical law
_____ 10. Patient-Care Partnership (Patient's Bill of Rights)
_____ 11. Patient Self-Determination Act
_____ 12. Confidentiality

a. gives medical authority to one person
b. study of genes
c. extraordinary care instructions
d. basic guidelines for hospital care
e. standards set by elected officials
f. federal law on extraordinary care
g. the medical ethics of moral issues
h. advanced means of replacing genes
i. maintaining secret patient information
j. principles governing medical conduct
k. counseling related to gene disorders
l. not to prolong life through extraordinary means

Chapter Review

1. What is the difference between medical ethics and medical law?

_____
_____
_____
_____

2. Why do medical associations develop statements of ethics?

_____
_____
_____
_____

3. Every physician must take the Hippocratic Oath. Why is this oath important?

_____
_____
_____
_____

4. Why are the Patient-Care Partnership, the Patient Self-Determination Act, and similar reforms important to medicine?

_____

_____

_____

_____

5. How and why is medical practice related to social policy?

_____

_____

_____

_____

6. Discuss what is meant by allocation of limited resources in medicine and name some of the important limited resources.

_____

_____

_____

_____

7. Why is prolonging life for terminally ill patients such a difficult issue for physicians?

_____

_____

_____

_____

8. What are some of the abuses of confidentiality that result from the use of computers?

_____

_____

_____

_____

9. What is the medical assistant's role in ethical issues?

_____

_____

_____

_____

10. How can a medical assistant contribute to maintaining confidentiality of patient records?

_____

_____

_____

_____

Critical Thinking Scenarios

1. A young woman is critically injured in an automobile accident and never regains consciousness. Because she does not have a living will, she is kept alive in a vegetative state for many years after her parents went to court to force doctors to maintain her on life support. Her husband says that he and his wife had discussed life and death matters many times and she had told him that she would never want to be kept on life support indefinitely. How do you think this matter should be handled?

_____

_____

_____

_____

2. After taking a position at Horseman and Winfield Obstetrics and Gynecology, P.C., you discover that both Dr. Horseman and Dr. Winfield are avidly pro-choice. It is very difficult for you, who are pro-life, to listen to their frequent and forceful opinions about the importance of abortion. You have never shared your viewpoint with the physicians? What will you do?

_____

_____

_____

_____

3. A young man suffering from a rare form of cancer is unable to receive a trial drug because his insurance policy does not cover the cost of the drug and he cannot afford the expense himself. As a medical assistant who understands that insurance companies must make money, what is your position?

_____

_____

_____

_____

4. At 32, your brother has been diagnosed with Parkinson's disease. Fetal stem cell research might lead to a cure in time to benefit your brother, yet you have previously believed that to create a fetus, harvest the stem cells, and then destroy the fetus is wrong. How does your brother's diagnosis affect your thinking?

_____

_____

_____

_____

5. You are at risk of a disastrous inherited disease that usually kills within ten years of being diagnosed. The disease can be detected through genetic testing, yet you are struggling with the decision of whether to be tested. You are not sure you want to know whether you carry the gene for the disease. What will you do?

_____

_____

_____

_____

6. The cardiology surgery practice where you work as a medical assistant has two patients waiting for a donor heart: one is a disabled 69-year-old man who is in remission for cancer, and the other is a 35-year-old mom with three small children. Neither may live more than six months without a transplant. The man is No. 1 on the transplant list in your area and the woman is No. 2. The story has hit the local newspaper and a great deal of controversy has erupted. What is your opinion?

_____

_____

_____

_____

7. The internal medicine specialist for whom you work as a medical assistant routinely refers patients to his brother, a psychiatrist. You often wonder whether so many of your patients really need psychiatric care. The number of referrals is beginning to disturb you. Do you have a responsibility in this situation? If so, what is your responsibility?

_____

_____

_____

_____

8. Three levels of charges are standard at Lowness and Barber, the practice where you work as a medical assistant: $55 for a brief visit, $70 for an intermediate visit, and $85 for an advanced visit. As costs of malpractice insurance have risen, you have noticed that your physician employer rarely labels a visit as brief. Consequently, patients now get charged the intermediate visit fee and advanced visit fee for the same amount of time that was called a basic visit previously. Do you have a responsibility in this situation? Why or why not?

_____

_____

_____

_____

9. You overhear the following conversation between the parents of a small child as they walk out the door of the practice where you are employed. After the family leaves, you hear the examining physician talking to a nurse about the child's suspicious bruises. Do you have a responsibility in this situation? If so, what is your responsibility?

   Mom: "I told them she fell off the swing set. I think it's okay. But I'm really mad about what you did."
   Dad: "Leave me alone. I don't want to talk about it."

_____

_____

_____

_____

10. Another medical assistant at Sholatz and Meyerstein makes the following comment. How will you respond?

   "Dr. Sholatz's son, Eric, got in trouble at school today. I took the call from the principal, who had to identify himself because Dr. Sholatz was with a patient. The principal said the call was urgent and wanted me to interrupt the doctor if possible. I hung around outside the door, and I heard Dr. Sholatz ask how long Eric would be expelled."

_____

_____

_____

_____

Simulation 3

Today is your third day of work at Marks and Graupera. Process today's papers according to the procedures you followed for previous simulations.

Supplies Needed

E-mail form
Blank paper
Notepaper
To Do List
Work Summary

Action Options, Suggestions, and Conflicts

- Your office is identical to the office shown in the Administrative CD. View the CD any time a reference is made to your office.
- Identify a spot in the office where you would want to hang the frame in Action Paper 3-2.
- Use a word processor to create any documents to be printed.

Action Paper 3-1

Marks and Graupera, P.C.

Note from Lydia

Look at your office area and determine whether there is anything that will interfere with maintaining confidentiality. I'd like you to make several recommendations about how we can heighten confidentiality around your desk. Just jot your thoughts down on this note and return it. Use the CD as a guide.

Action Paper 3-2

Marks and Graupera, P.C.

Note from Tarik

Here is my old copy of the AAMA Code of Ethics. When you get a chance, you should key and print a copy for your office. It has always helped me focus on the right thing to do. Let me know where you want to hang the Code, and I'll help you frame and put it up.

T. L.

Name: _____   Date: _____

To: Your name@MarksandGraupera.com
From: Luke Streeter@MarksandGraupera.com
Subject: AAMA meeting

Dr. Marks and Dr. Graupera would like you to join the local AAMA chapter. I've been a member for six years. The next meeting is three weeks away—August 14. Why don't you attend as my guest?

The subject is medical ethics. We're each to bring two questions we have about issues in medical ethics. E-mail me your questions after you decide what you want to ask.

Action Paper 3-4

Dr. Graupera: "(your name), will you come into my office, please."

You: "Of course."

Dr. Graupera: "Our office holds all employees to the highest ethical standards. One of the reasons we felt you would fit in so well here is that I sense you, too, are a very ethical person. I would like you to give me your opinion of the biggest issues facing medical assistants who work in a small medical office."

You:

_____

_____

_____

_____

Name: _____ Date: _____

To Do List

-

-

-

-

-

-

-

-

-

-

-

-

-

-

-

-

Name: _____

Date Started: _____ Date Completed: _____

Work Summary 3

Section 1

1. Record the numbers of the Action Papers marked "Rush."　　_____

2. Record the numbers of the Action Papers marked "ASAP."　　_____

3. Record the numbers of the Action Papers marked "Routine."　　_____

Section 2

4. Write the list of "To Do" items and the actions that were taken. When this section is complete, turn the Work Summary over to your instructor, who will evaluate your work and return it for your later use.

To Do   Action Taken

_____   _____

_____   _____

_____   _____

_____   _____

_____   _____

_____   _____

Section 3

5. You will receive two assessments for your work—one is based on time to complete the items and the other is based on quality of work. Your instructor will complete the Assessment portion of the Work Summary.

Points Received

Time Required   _____

　　　　　20 points   25 minutes or less
　　　　　15 points   30 minutes
　　　　　10 points   35 minutes
　　　　　 5 points   40 minutes

Quality of Work   _____

Total Points _____

CHAPTER 4
Medical Law

Chapter Outline

Key Vocabulary Terms

Match each word or term with its correct meaning.

_____ 1. Advance directives

_____ 2. Civil law

_____ 3. Criminal law

_____ 4. Drug schedules

_____ 5. Good Samaritan laws

_____ 6. Informed consent

_____ 7. Malfeasance

_____ 8. Misfeasance

_____ 9. Nonfeasance

a. failure to act when duty requires

b. drug categories divided according to abuse potential

c. lawful treatment performed in the wrong way

d. laws protecting physicians in emergency situations

e. wrongful treatment of a patient

f. rights and obligations one has toward society

g. a patient's right to medical information about risk

h. rights and obligations of one person toward another

i. a patient's wishes regarding future treatment

Chapter Review

1. What factors have contributed to medical laws becoming more complicated and controversial?

_____

_____

_____

_____

2. What is the purpose of the Medical Practices Act?

_____

_____

_____

_____

3. What are the purposes of licensure?

_____

_____

_____

_____

_____

_____

4. For what reasons can a physician's license be revoked or suspended?

_____

_____

_____

_____

5. How can a medical assistant help a physician in matters related to the law?

_____

_____

_____

_____

6. What are the two divisions of law and what do they govern?

_____

_____

_____

7. Discuss the concept of negligence and the three types of negligence. Give an example of each.

_____

_____

_____

_____

8. What are the physician's responsibilities under the concept of material risk?

_____

_____

_____

_____

9. In what ways does a physician rely on the medical assistant regarding informed consent?

_____

_____

_____

_____

10. What does the legal concept of privilege of patient confidentiality guarantee?

_____

_____

_____

_____

Critical Thinking Scenarios

1. A fellow medical assistant at Holgood and Marks Neurological Associates was fired last week for what the physician explained was "good cause." She calls you at home to say she is planning to file a complaint with a state oversight agency because she did not have due process of law. Although you refrained from discussing the issue with her, you have an opinion about her ability to prevail in an action. What is your opinion?

_____

_____

_____

_____

2. Tarik is worried because a friend of his, also a clinical medical assistant, has been sued for malpractice because he gave a patient incorrect instructions after misinterpreting the physician's comments. Tarik does not have professional liability coverage and says he cannot afford to purchase the insurance. He asks what you think.

_____

_____

_____

_____

3. Sarah Annenberg, 44 years old, is excited about her first pregnancy. The OB/GYN finds her in excellent health and assures her that a return visit is not necessary for two months. When she miscarries one month later, she is angry with the doctor for not scheduling her more often. She hinted to you that she might sue for malpractice, and you wonder what form of negligence she might identify in her suit. What do you decide and what are your reasons?

_____

_____

_____

_____

4. A father brings his 8-year-old son to Bradbury & Wayne Internal Medicine and Surgery after the child complains of pain in his side. Dr. Wayne diagnoses appendicitis, then instructs you to schedule the child for immediate surgery and to prepare the informed consent forms. Because the child is crying and appears to be in great pain, you are distracted as you gather the forms and give them to the father to sign. Later, as you are filing the documents in the patient's record, you discover a missing form. Dr. Wayne has already left for the hospital, and the surgery is scheduled in thirty minutes. You are sure Dr. Wayne will be annoyed with you if you call and tell him a form is missing. What will you do?

_____

_____

_____

_____

5. You overhear a conversation between Dr. Anton and a patient who happens to be your father's boss. Dr. Anton is telling the patient that he has prostate cancer. You know your dad will be disappointed if you have this information but do not tell him. What will you do?

_____

_____

_____

_____

6. Rumor among your friends is that Shana, a former classmate who is a patient at your practice, has a history of drug abuse. From her medical record, you learn that she is HIV positive. You make the mistake of telling your best friend that you saw Shana, and your friend assumes you saw her at work. She asks you what is wrong with Shana. You realize you have made a mistake by sharing information and think about saying that you ran into Shana at lunch. However, you and your friend have promised never to lie to each other. What will you do?

_____

_____

_____

_____

7. Ralph Tamiki was given written notice by certified mail, return receipt requested, that the physicians in your practice will no longer treat him because he was noncompliant about taking his medications and keeping appointments. The patient calls and demands an appointment. He says he never received the letter, and he comments, "You're going to hear from my lawyer if you don't give me an appointment." What will you do?

_____

_____

_____

_____

8. A 6-year-old patient at Moro and Pasinelli Pediatric Associates whom the doctor diagnosed with a broken arm whispers to you, "My mom hit me with her tennis racquet." What will you do?

_____

_____

_____

_____

9. A businessman rushes into the doctor's office fifteen minutes late for his annual physical and says, "I need to fax something to my office right away. May I come inside to your desk and send this form to my secretary?" How will you respond?

_____

_____

_____

_____

10. A local television celebrity is a patient of one of the physicians in your group. Although you rarely work with this doctor, you are really curious about why the patient came in. You would like to access the patient's record, and you have no intention of sharing anything you learn. You think the best time to look at the record is when the office is busy and the other staff members are distracted. What will you do?

_____

_____

_____

_____

Simulation 4

Today is your fourth day of work at Marks and Graupera. You are on your own.

Supplies Needed
Four sheets of blank paper
To Do List
Work Summary

Action Options, Suggestions, and Conflicts
• Use a word processor to create any documents to be printed.
• Write or print directly on the Action Paper, when appropriate.

Name: _____   Date: _____

Action Paper 4-1

To: Your name@MarksandGraupera.com
From: LydiaMakay@aol.com
Subject: Task list

Dr. Graupera asked me to develop some statistics for a talk he's giving on medical malpractice for the local AAMA chapter and I'm late with it. Will you do the following for me, please?

1. Locate statistics on malpractice claims by specialty and prioritize them in descending order.

2. Key and print the list for Dr. Graupera so he can hand it out at his talk. By the end of the week, I'll need to add this to his PowerPoint presentation.

Action Paper 4-2

Caller: Hello. Who is this?

You: This is (your name). I am the medical assistant. May I ask who's calling?

Caller: This is Madge West. Someone at your office gave me some advance forms to fill out before my surgery and told me to take them to the hospital with me.

You: Yes, I know the forms you're talking about. They're called the advance directives.

Caller: Well, I don't think I'm going to sign them. What they say scares me.

You:

Caller: Well, the forms talk about dying, and the doctor said this surgery was not life-threatening.

You:

Caller: Well, I want Dr. Graupera to call me.

You:

Action Paper 4-3

Dr. Graupera: "Lydia tells me you're helping her with my talk for the AAMA chapter. Here are a few notes I've made about the medical assistant's role in obtaining consent. Will you add a few procedures that a medical assistant can follow to ensure that consent has been obtained, then key and print the sheet for me? Make it look nice, please."

You: "Thanks, Dr. G."

Dr. Graupera: "Oh, give a copy to Lydia, too, so she can keep track of everything that will go into my presentation."

Informed Consent

Protect yourself! Make sure your staff is fully knowledgeable about informed consent. Patients often ask the staff questions they're reluctant to ask the physician. While the staff should be directed to refer all such questions to the physician, they should understand informed consent.

Make sure all staff recognizes the extreme importance of having properly executed informed consent documents in cases where they are needed The medical assistants, especially, are important in obtaining consent before a procedure is performed. I'm providing a list of guidelines every medical assistant should follow regarding informed consent. I recommend that you duplicate it and give a copy to each medical assistant in your offices.

Action Paper 4-4

Please read Dr. Marks's note. Will you prepare the rough draft of a new letter for me? I'll edit it and give it back to you for corrections.
Lydia

Marks and Graupera, P.C.

Note from Dr. Marks

Lydia, I've been looking over our current physician withdrawal letter and find it to be incomplete. It is far too brief and doesn't cover the essentials needed these days. We need to take care of this right away, so I'd like to see a new version by tomorrow afternoon. Put something together for me to review. I'm sure you can find a sample on the AAMA or AMA Internet site.

Action Paper 4-5

Note from Tarik

There's a crossword puzzle about ethical and legal matters on our office CD that I gave you. Why don't you work on it when you get a chance. It's fun.

Name: _____   Date: _____

To Do List

-
-
-
-
-
-
-
-
-
-
-
-
-
-
-
-
-

Name: _____

Date Started: _____ Date Completed: _____

Work Summary 4

Section 1

1. Record the numbers of the Action Papers marked "Rush." _____

2. Record the numbers of the Action Papers marked "ASAP." _____

3. Record the numbers of the Action Papers marked "Routine." _____

Section 2

4. Write the list of "To Do" items and the actions that were taken. When this section is complete, turn the Work Summary over to your instructor, who will evaluate your work and return it for your later use.

To Do | Action Taken

_____ _____

_____ _____

_____ _____

_____ _____

_____ _____

_____ _____

Section 3

5. You will receive two assessments for your work—one is based on time to complete the items and the other is based on quality of work. Your instructor will complete the Assessment portion of the Work Summary.

Points Received

Time Required

               20 points   70 minutes or less   _____

               15 points   100 minutes

               10 points   130 minutes

                 5 points   160 minutes

Quality of Work   _____

Total Points _____

PART II Patient Relations

CHAPTER 5
Interacting with Patients

Chapter Outline

Interpersonal Communication
      Concern for the Patient
      Listening
      Empathy
      Tact
      Patience
Importance of Verbal and Nonverbal Communication
      Verbal Communication
      Nonverbal Communication
      Feedback
Computers and Relationships with Patients
Managing Patient Activities
      Managing the Reception Area or Lobby
            Reception Area Appearance
            Orderly Flow of Patient Traffic
      Greeting Patients
            Established Patients
            New Patients
Discussing Finances and Billing
      Importance of the First Visit
      Insurance Company Payments
Handling Emergencies
      Recognizing an Emergency
      Obtaining Specific Information about Call-in Emergency Patients
      Arranging for Emergency Medical Care
      Reassuring Family and Waiting Patients
Chapter Activities
      Performance-Based Activities
      Expanding Your Thinking

Key Vocabulary Terms

Match each word or term with its correct meaning.

_____ 1. Active listening

_____ 2. Empathy

_____ 3. Feedback

_____ 4. Interpersonal

_____ 5. Nonverbal communication

_____ 6. Tact

a. diplomacy in handling difficult situations

b. from one person to another

c. paying conscious attention to the speaker

d. can include facial expressions and gestures

e. responses that provide direction

f. mentally putting oneself in another's place

Chapter Review

1. What is meant by the term "interpersonal communication"?

   _____

   _____

   _____

   _____

2. Name and describe several behaviors necessary for good interpersonal communication.

   _____

   _____

   _____

   _____

   _____

   _____

   _____

   _____

3. Give an example of a verbal message and a nonverbal message that might seem contradictory to a patient.

   _____

   _____

   _____

   _____

   _____

4. Name several examples of nonverbal communication that a medical assistant might use during a typical day.

   _____

   _____

   _____

   _____

5. Why is patient feedback important during a conversation?

   _____

   _____

   _____

   _____

6. Why is eye contact important when talking with patients?

_____

_____

_____

_____

7. What can a medical assistant do to ensure that the lobby is comfortable for waiting patients?

_____

_____

_____

_____

8. In what ways should a new patient and an established patient be treated differently?

_____

_____

_____

_____

9. What items of information should be obtained during an emergency call?

_____

_____

_____

_____

10. List several medical emergencies that should be clearly apparent to a medical assistant.

_____

_____

_____

_____

Critical Thinking Scenarios

1. You are surprised when the physician tells you that Mrs. Rainier, 75 years old, complained that you were rude and ignored her when she signed in. You explain that you tried to answer all of Mrs. Rainier's questions but that she kept interrupting when you were trying to get a report out for the billing clerk. The doctor replies that this is not the first time patients have mentioned that they felt ignored. What might you be doing to give this impression to patients?

   _____

   _____

   _____

   _____

2. A woman cries softly as she waits in the lobby for her husband to return from the oncologist's examination. The other patients appear anxious when her sobbing increases. What should you do?

   _____

   _____

   _____

   _____

3. Mrs. Abjay's sensitivity radar increases when she visits the doctor. She becomes anxious and her blood pressure leaps. She experiences the "white coat syndrome." What will you do to relieve her anxiety?

   _____

   _____

   _____

   _____

4. An angry, irritable patient loudly questions every charge on his bill and complains about how much he is being required to pay. What will you say to this patient?

   _____

   _____

   _____

   _____

5. You notice that a patient looks flushed, strained, and tense. When you ask whether she is ill, she nervously says, "No." The extroverted patient next to her tries several times to start a conversation, and the woman rejects her attempts. What could you do to help her?

_____

_____

_____

_____

6. Hans Meier walks with a cane after an automobile accident that amputated his right leg. He moves slowly and with great difficulty. Because he is a big man, he takes a large part of the hallway as he moves along, and this interferes with other patient traffic. When you are busy, you find his slow progress frustrating. You try not to appear impatient, yet it is hard for you. How should you handle this situation?

_____

_____

_____

_____

7. Samuel Cooper has been a patient for several years. He often brings candy for the staff, and he likes to stay around after his appointment to talk with you. This is a problem when you have several tasks to accomplish. How might you handle the situation?

_____

_____

_____

_____

8. People often tell you to smile or ask why you are frowning. Occasionally, they ask whether everything is okay with you. Normally, you answer, "I'm smiling on the inside," or "I'm great." You do not understand why they misunderstand your demeanor. What can you do?

_____

_____

_____

_____

9. The office manager says to you, "You need to sound more pleasant on the phone. Patients are misunderstanding your efficiency for curtness." What can you do?

_____

_____

_____

_____

10. A woman brings her son who is bleeding from his mouth into the main lobby. One patient gasps and several others stand up to help. How will you handle this situation?

_____

_____

_____

_____

Simulation 5

Today is your fifth day of work at Marks and Graupera. Make decisions regarding the actions to be taken.

Supplies Needed

Blank paper
Telephone log
To Do List
Work Summary

Action Options, Suggestions, and Conflicts

- Follow the pattern of the simulated conversations in the textbook to fill in your part of the telephone and face-to-face conversations. Write directly on each Action Paper. For the telephone log, make up any information that is missing.

Action Paper 5-1

You, to a registering patient: "Good morning, I'll be with you in just a moment. Would you like to have a seat?"

Patient, after a while: "I've been waiting five minutes. Don't you want my name?"

You:

Action Paper 5-2

Marks and Graupera, P.C.

Note from Lydia

The lobby has seemed cluttered lately. Please give me a plan for keeping it more organized and attractive.

Action Paper 5-3

Time: 9:02 AM

Caller: This is Laisa Iman. I have an emergency (followed by several garbled words).

You:

Caller: Please get the doctor on the phone.

You (realizing the physician is examining another patient):

Caller: I said this is an emergency. I don't want to talk to an assistant.

You:

Caller: My husband has been vomiting blood since last night. He can't stand up without falling.

You:

Action Paper 5-4

Marks and Graupera, P.C.

Note from Judith Marks

Thanks for your fast actions this morning when the heart attack victim's wife brought him here instead of going directly to the hospital. Since you open for us each day, I guess we should have assumed that one day you would be confronted with such a situation, but I am sorry you were alone to deal with this problem. For the patient's record, I need a complete summary of how you handled this emergency.

Patient: "Isn't that the minister's wife with Dr. Graupera?"

You: "Yes, that is Mrs. Winfield."

Patient: "What's wrong with her?"

You:

Patient: "You can tell me. I would never tell anyone else."

You:

Patient: "I don't think she looks well. Has she been sick a long time?"

You:

Action Paper 5-6

Note from Lydia

Please refer to the telephone log shown on our office CD to list all of the incoming calls you take.

Received Time By	Patient's Name	Telephone No.	Reason for Call	Call Returned
_____	_____	_____	_____	_____
_____	_____	_____	_____	_____
_____	_____	_____	_____	_____
_____	_____	_____	_____	_____
_____	_____	_____	_____	_____
_____	_____	_____	_____	_____
_____	_____	_____	_____	_____
_____	_____	_____	_____	_____
_____	_____	_____	_____	_____
_____	_____	_____	_____	_____

Name: _____ Date: _____

To Do List

-
-
-
-
-
-
-
-
-
-
-
-
-
-
-
-

Name: _____

Date Started: _____ Date Completed: _____

Work Summary 5

Section 1

1. Record the numbers of the Action Papers marked "Rush."   _____

2. Record the numbers of the Action Papers marked "ASAP."   _____

3. Record the numbers of the Action Papers marked "Routine." _____

Section 2

4. Write the list of "To Do" items and the actions that were taken. When this section is complete, turn the Work Summary over to your instructor, who will evaluate your work and return it for your later use.

To Do   Action Taken

_____   _____

_____   _____

_____   _____

_____   _____

_____   _____

_____   _____

Section 3

5. You will receive two assessments for your work—one is based on time to complete the items and the other is based on quality of work. Your instructor will complete the Assessment portion of the Work Summary.

Points Received

Time Required   _____

          20 points   35 minutes or less
          15 points   40 minutes
          10 points   45 minutes
          5 points   50 minutes

Quality of Work   _____

Total Points _____

CHAPTER 6
Telecommunications

Chapter Outline

Key Vocabulary Terms

Match each word or term with its correct meaning.

_____ 1. Answering service   a. collect call

_____ 2. Cellular phone   b. twenty-four-hour phone answering service

_____ 3. DDD   c. function that allows a call to wait on the line

_____ 4. E-mail   d. call evaluation

_____ 5. Fax   e. electronic mail

_____ 6. Hold   f. message that requires a return call

_____ 7. Modem   g. geographic area identified by time of day

_____ 8. Reversed charges   h. conference via telephone, video, and computer

_____ 9. Screening   i. voice messages left on an answering machine

_____ 10. Time zone   j. Direct Distance Dialing

_____ 11. Callback   k. single call connecting several individuals

_____ 12. Conference call   l. portable phone

_____ 13. Videoconference   m. connects computers via the phone line

_____ 14. Voice mail   n. facsimile transmission of documents

Chapter Review

1. Discuss two telephone answering behaviors that annoy patients.

_____

_____

_____

_____

2. Explain the proper method of using the "hold" function.

_____

_____

_____

_____

3. Under what circumstances should long-distance calls be placed person-to-person?

_____

_____

_____

_____

4. Describe the procedure for screening calls.

_____

_____

_____

_____

5. Under what circumstances should a collect call be taken?

_____

_____

_____

_____

6. What is the importance of time zones when making long-distance calls?

_____

_____

_____

7. What is the purpose of the yellow pages and blue pages of a telephone directory?

_____

_____

_____

_____

8. What general rule should be followed regarding when to interrupt a physician by using a pager or cell phone?

_____

_____

_____

_____

9. How have telecommunications improved patient care?

_____

_____

_____

_____

10. What can a medical assistant do to reduce the negative effect of an answering machine greeting?

_____

_____

_____

_____

Critical Thinking Scenarios

1. Dr. Ebrez is always available by pager, even at the hospital where she is currently making rounds. Her tennis partner, who is leaving for an appointment, calls and asks whether Dr. Ebrez can play after work today. He needs to reserve a court. What should you do?

_____

_____

_____

_____

2. You are busy finalizing the checkout procedure for a patient who has finished her appointment when another patient calls and asks to hold until you can locate insurance information in her file. What should you do?

_____

_____

_____

_____

3. A person who identifies himself as an old family friend visiting in town for a "couple of hours" asks to talk to the physician. The doctor is examining one patient and has a waiting room full of other patients. How should you handle this call?

_____

_____

_____

_____

4. The physician's daughter who attends boarding school in another state calls while the physician is examining a patient. How should you handle this call?

_____

_____

_____

_____

5. You receive a collect call from a former patient who now lives in another city. She had changed from your physician to another before she left your town. Should you take the collect call? Explain your reasoning.

_____

_____

_____

_____

6. A voice that is vaguely familiar asks to speak to the physician, saying that the call is "important." When you ask who is calling, the caller says, "It's personal." It could be a patient, one of the physician's friends, or a salesperson. How should you handle this call?

_____

_____

_____

_____

7. A patient who is visiting in California calls your office in Charleston, South Carolina, where it is 1 PM, and asks you to have the doctor call her before she catches a plane at 5 PM. You do not discuss whether she means 5 PM in California or in Charleston. To be safe, by what time should the physician return the call?

_____

_____

_____

_____

8. You seem to be having difficulty finding the telephone number for Canella St. Rodes in the directory. In fact, you are surprised that there are no names starting with "St." How will you locate the name?

_____

_____

_____

_____

9. One of your responsibilities as office manager at Floberg and Rinestein, P.C. is to recommend services needed by the practice. Lately, you have noticed problems with the answering machine. Because the machine is several years old, you consider replacing it with voice mail from your telephone carrier, but another medical assistant tells you he thinks this is a bad idea. What reasons make voice mail an attractive option for the office?

_____

_____

_____

_____

10. The physician is making rounds at the hospital, yet you need to reach him about a very sick patient who has come to the office without an appointment. Should you use the physician's cell phone or beeper to reach him?

_____

_____

_____

_____

Simulation 6

Today is your sixth day of work at Marks and Graupera.

Supplies Needed

Three telephone message forms
Two telephone script forms
To Do List
Work Summary

Action Options, Suggestions, and Conflicts

• When information for callback messages is given, interpret the information and transfer it to a callback form.

• If asked to make a call for one of the physicians, fill in a telephone script form.

Name: _____   Date: _____

Marks and Graupera, P.C.

Note from Lydia

Dr. Graupera needs to set up a conference call with two consulting physicians and Magadlina Malta, his patient, this afternoon. The doctors are expecting the call; however, there is the possibility that they will have been called away for an emergency. Therefore, call the physicians directly instead of calling just their office. Ms. Malta is here in Philadelphia; Dr. Randell is in Houston; Dr. Sinchita is in Denver; and Dr. Alamin is in Nashville. Make the arrangements for the conference call and leave me a note telling me what time you want Dr. Graupera to be available.

On second thought, since this is your first conference call for us, write out your plan for setting up the call and give it to me first for approval.

Name: _____ Date: _____

Action Paper 6-2

To: Your name@MarksandGraupera.com
From: LydiaMakay@MarksandGraupera.com
Subject: Telephone greeting

Here is a transcript of our telephone greetings. I think we need to update the greetings and make them more cordial. Will you edit the greetings? Thanks.

Greeting 1: Good morning, this is the office of Dr. Judith; Marks and Dr. Ramon Graupera, (name of person answering) speaking. How may I help you?

Greeting 2: Marks and Graupera, P.C., hold please.

Greeting 3: Good morning, this is (name of person speaking). You have reached the doctors' offices. May I ask which doctor you would like to speak with?

Name: _____ Date: _____

Action Paper 6-3

Marks and Graupera, P.C.

Note from Tarik

Help! I have to make a presentation on telephone etiquette at next month's AAMA meeting. Will you make a list of the things you think I should cover and give me some pointers on good telephone answering techniques?

Thanks.

Action Paper 6-4a

Callback information for Dr. Graupera

Message 1: 11 AM, today—RX Health Days called with a question on the prescription for Jason Berkim. Dr. Graupera ordered phenylephrine nose drops for Jason, but the writing is not clear. Should he have two drops or three drops in each nostril? Also, does the message mean that he's to have the drops fifteen to twenty minutes before bedtime, or is that fifteen to twenty minutes before dinnertime?

Message 2: 11:45 AM today—Marcus Boatmeyer called. His daughter, Andrea, had a fever and stomachache all day yesterday and last night, and she vomited several times last night. He wants to know what medicine he can give her. He says if Dr. Graupera is not in he's willing to take the advice of the medical assistant.

Message 3: 2 PM—Dr. Marks's attorney called and wants to set up an appointment for one day this week. He will make himself available on Dr. Marks's schedule. She should call back with the date and time she wants to come in. The meeting is about the malpractice suit Mr. Adelaide has filed.

NAME			PHONE / EXAM	DX			
DATE	TIME	DR					
FROM TO				RETURN PHONE # WILL CALL BACK		RETURN TIME	TELEPHONE CONVERSATION RECORD
MESSAGE CC/HC							PHARMACY
							PHONE ❑ AGE WT
							AMT
							SIG _____
							FOR _____
							SIDE EFFECTS ____ REFILL
							FOLLOW UP

Name: _____ Date: _____

Action Paper 6-4b

NAME			PHONE / EXAM	DX		
DATE	TIME	DR				

FROM TO		RETURN PHONE # WILL CALL BACK	RETURN TIME	TELEPHONE CONVERSATION RECORD

MESSAGE CC/HC _____

_____

_____

_____

_____

_____

_____

_____

_____

_____

_____

_____

_____

_____

PHARMACY

PHONE ☐   AGE WT

AMT

SIG _____

FOR _____

SIDE EFFECTS _____ REFILL

FOLLOW UP

NAME			PHONE / EXAM	DX		
DATE	TIME	DR				

FROM TO		RETURN PHONE # WILL CALL BACK	RETURN TIME	TELEPHONE CONVERSATION RECORD

MESSAGE CC/HC _____

_____

_____

_____

_____

_____

_____

_____

_____

_____

_____

_____

_____

_____

PHARMACY

PHONE ☐   AGE WT

AMT

SIG _____

FOR _____

SIDE EFFECTS _____ REFILL

FOLLOW UP

Action Paper 6-5a

Marks and Graupera, P.C.

Note from Dr. Graupera

1. Please call General Hospital and make arrangements for admitting Susan Boyd today by 4 PM. Susan, who is 6 years old, needs an isolation room. Her diagnosis is scarlet fever. She should have complete bed rest, except for bathroom privileges and should eat only from the diabetic menu. I will leave further instructions when I make rounds. Dr. Manning will consult.

2. Please call the Boyd residence and confirm with Mr. or Mrs. Boyd the arrangements I made for Susan's admittance to General Hospital.

Telephone Script Form

You:

Second party:

You:

Second party:

You:

Second party:

You:

Second party:

You:

Second party:

You:

Second party:

You:

Second party:

You:

Second party:

You:

Second party:

You:

Second party:

Action Paper 6-5b

Telephone Script Form
You:
Second party:
You:
Second party:
You:
Second party:
You:
Second party:
You:
Second party:
You:
Second party:
You:
Second party:
You:
Second party:
You:
Second party:

Name: _____   Date: _____

Action Paper 6-6

Note from Lydia

As a reminder of good telephone etiquette, I'd like you to take the telephone quiz on our office CD.

Name: _____   Date: _____

To Do List

-

-

-

-

-

-

-

-

-

-

-

-

-

-

-

-

Name: _____

Date Started: _____ Date Completed: _____

Work Summary 6

Section 1

1. Record the numbers of the Action Papers marked "Rush." _____

2. Record the numbers of the Action Papers marked "ASAP." _____

3. Record the numbers of the Action Papers marked "Routine." _____

Section 2

4. Write the list of "To Do" items and the actions that were taken. When this section is complete, turn the Work Summary over to your instructor, who will evaluate your work and return it for your later use.

To Do   Action Taken

_____   _____

_____   _____

_____   _____

_____   _____

_____   _____

_____   _____

Section 3

5. You will receive two assessments for your work—one is based on time to complete the items and the other is based on quality of work. Your instructor will complete the Assessment portion of the Work Summary.

Points Received

Time Required   _____
    20 points   70 minutes or less
    15 points   90 minutes
    10 points   110 minutes
     5 points   130 minutes

Quality of Work   _____

                              Total Points _____

CHAPTER 7
Scheduling Appointments

Chapter Outline

Key Vocabulary Terms

Match each word or term with its correct meaning.

_____ 1. Allocation

_____ 2. Computer scheduling

_____ 3. Daily list of appointments

_____ 4. Effective

_____ 5. Efficient

_____ 6. Optimal

_____ 7. Overbooking

_____ 8. Progress appointments

_____ 9. Referral

_____ 10. Wave scheduling

_____ 11. Appointment book

_____ 12. No show

_____ 13. Schedule

_____ 14. Triage

a. clustering appointments by time block

b. serving patients without efficient resource handling

c. screening emergency calls

d. sending patient to a specialist

e. patient who fails to keep an appointment

f. too many patients in one time slot

g. list of patients being seen in one day

h. daily record of patient information

i. making good use of available resources

j. daily calendar of appointment times

k. follow-up appointments

l. making the best use of a resource

m. scheduling appointments with computer software

n. deciding how to divide available resources

Chapter Review

1. What factors should be taken into consideration when scheduling patients?

_____

_____

_____

_____

2. Explain the concept of cluster scheduling.

_____

_____

_____

_____

_____

_____

_____

_____

3. What is the difference between wave scheduling and modified wave scheduling?

_____

_____

_____

_____

_____

4. When doctors have "open hours," patients are seen on what type of schedule?

_____

_____

_____

_____

5. What questions might a medical assistant ask to determine a patient's medical condition before scheduling an appointment?

_____

_____

_____

_____

_____

6. In scheduling, what is meant by the term "double tracking"?

_____

_____

_____

7. How is a canceled appointment handled in the appointment book?

_____

_____

_____

_____

8. What common reasons cause a medical office to get behind schedule?

_____

_____

_____

_____

9. How should missed appointments be handled in the appointment book?

_____

_____

_____

_____

10. What information should be provided on the daily list of appointments?

_____

_____

_____

_____

Critical Thinking Scenarios

1. Dr. Tambulo, the obstetrician for whom you work, calls from the hospital at 8:30 AM to say he has scheduled an emergency C-section and will not be in until 10:30. The appointment book is heavily scheduled and the first two patients arrive as you are talking with Dr. Tambulo. How will you handle this situation?

_____

_____

_____

_____

2. Dr. Suk has fallen forty-five minutes behind schedule, and the lobby is filling with fidgety patients who frequently ask you, "How much longer before I get to see the doctor?" What should you do?

_____

_____

_____

_____

3. One of the patients is notorious for missing his appointments and calling later to apologize and reschedule. How should you handle this situation?

_____

_____

_____

_____

4. A salesperson arrives at the office shortly after lunch and asks to see the physician. You are knowledgeable about the product the salesperson represents and are sure the physician will not want to talk with her, so you do not schedule an appointment. The salesperson is insistent, saying she will wait until the doctor is free. How will you handle this situation?

_____

_____

_____

_____

5. A patient with a cough, a scratchy voice, and watering eyes walks in without an appointment. What will you do?

_____

_____

_____

_____

6. Dr. Vazquez walks to your desk with a patient and says that he is referring the patient to Dr. Weir. He asks you to give the patient the information she needs. What information will you provide?

_____

_____

_____

_____

7. Anna Srouji calls to say she needs to come in for an appointment immediately. She thinks she has appendicitis. What questions will you ask Anna?

_____

_____

_____

_____

8. You notice that someone crossed out time in the appointment book without writing the purpose of the time out. What assumption could you make about why the time was crossed out?

_____

_____

_____

_____

9. Dr. Severson tells you that she will be on vacation the weeks of February 10, May 9, September 14, and November 25. What action should you take immediately?

_____

_____

_____

_____

10. Dr. Concepcion Suarez alerts you that Donald Mouser is to be scheduled for the hospital. What information will you obtain from the patient's file before calling the hospital?

_____

_____

_____

_____

Simulation 7

Today is your seventh day of work at Marks and Graupera.

Supplies Needed

Appointment book page
To Do List
Work Summary

Action Options, Suggestions, and Conflicts

- Read Action Papers 7-1 through 7-7.
- Schedule all appointments on the Appointment book page provided.

Name: _____ Date: _____

MEMO FROM
DR. RAMON GRAUPERA

Please schedule a consultation appointment for Leslie Roland on July 17, so I can review the results of his CPE. He needs an early a.m. or late p.m. appointment.

RG

Name: _____ Date: _____

DATE **7/15/—**

TO **Dr. Graupera's Secretary**   TIME **9:00 a.m.**

TELEPHONE MESSAGE

M **rs. Nancy Armand** OF _____

ADDRESS _____

CALLED	✓	WANTS TO SEE YOU		RETURNED YOUR CALL	
PLEASE CALL	✓	WILL CALL AGAIN		URGENT	

MESSAGE **Cancelled her 3:30 appt. today. Wants to reschedule for 7/17 at 3:30. Please change the appointment. Call her if change cannot be made.**

PHONE NUMBER **565-6868**   TAKEN BY **Tina**

Name: _____ Date: _____

TELEPHONE MESSAGE	
DATE _7/15/–_ TIME _9:30 a.m._ DR. _Graupera_ NAME _Mrs. Waasdorp_ PATIENT'S NAME _Sandy Waasdorp_ ☐ TELEPHONED RETURN PHONE NO. _____ RETURN TIME _____ ☐ WILL CALL BACK TO _Dr. Graupera's secretary_ FROM _Victoria Ramonez_	PHARMACY _____ PHONE _____ AGE _____ WT. _____
MESSAGE _____ _Sandy Waasdorp will not be in at 3:30 p.m. tomorrow for her checkup. Ms. Waasdorp has resheduled the appointment for July 17 at 2:00 p.m. You need to make the changes in the appoinment book. I confirmed the time with Ms. Waasdorp._ _Rolff_	PRESCRIPTION STRENGTH _____ AMOUNT _____ LABEL _____ _____ _____ FOR _____ ☐ SIDE EFFECTS ___ REFILL FOLLOW-UP_____ _____ _____

DATE	7/15/–
TO _Dr. Graupera's Secretary_	TIME	10:30 a.m.

TELEPHONE MESSAGE

M _rs. Abernathy, secretary_ OF _Dr. Linda Bronner's office_

ADDRESS _____

CALLED	✓	WANTS TO SEE YOU		RETURNED YOUR CALL	
PLEASE CALL		WILL CALL AGAIN		URGENT	

MESSAGE _Dr. Bronner is referring Mrs. Sally Fields to Dr. Graupera for a consultation. Make an appointment for Mrs. Fields for 7/16 or 7/17; then call Mrs. Fields and tell her the date and time._

PHONE NUMBER 555-1283   TAKEN BY _Jose_

Action Paper 7-5

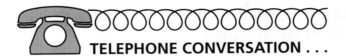

TELEPHONE CONVERSATION . . .

Telephone rings

Medical Secretary:	Good morning. Dr. Graupera's office. May I help you?
Patient:	This is Walter Burgham. We are going out of town Thursday. I would like to come into the office Tuesday afternoon or Wednesday morning for a recheck of my strep throat. Is that possible?
Medical Secretary:	I'll check the appointment book. One moment please. (Pause) Dr. Graupera can see you at 2:45 P.M. Tuesday or between 9 and 10 A.M. Wednesday. Which time is more convenient for you?
Patient:	May I come in Tuesday at 3:30 instead of 2:45?

Action Paper 7-6

MEMO FROM
DR. RAMON GRAUPERA

July 16, 20--

Sheila Duckworth of Medical Micrographics, Inc., would like to demonstrate micrographics equipment to us on Wednesday, July 17. I have asked my new medical assistant to arrange my calendar, so I can see the demo at 4 p.m. and I would like you to attend also. We may soon lease micrographics equipment for our inactive medical records.

Name: _____   Date: _____

DESK NOTES

From: **Ramon Graupera, M.D.**

7/16

Scott Lansing, my attorney, needs to see me for about an hour on Wednesday. If there is an hour free immediately before or after lunch, make the appointment then. He will call you this morning for a confirmation.

RG

Name: _____ Date: _____

Action Paper 7-7b

| MONDAY | *July 15* | | TUESDAY | *July 16* | | WEDNESDAY | *July 17* |

MONDAY July 15

9	00	555-1419 — Matthew Jackson / Tired, can't sleep
	15	
	30	
	45	555-0010 — Martha McClendon / cash on hand /
10	00	
	15	555-6908
	30	John Roosevelt / Urinary problems
	45	
11	00	Richard Duncan / Checkup / SSS-3011
	15	Paul Roser / Sore throat / SSS-1281
	30	
	45	
12	00	Lunch
	15	
	30	
	45	
1	00	
	15	
	30	Complete — 555- — Leslie Roland / physical exam / 7010
	45	↓
2	00	
	15	Suzanne Cadle / Eye tearing / SSS-4391
	30	
	45	555-1192 — Barbara Bayer / Old knee injury /
3	00	
	15	
	30	Nancy Armand / Pap / SSS-6868
	45	
4	00	
	15	
	30	
	45	

TUESDAY July 16

9	00	Jane Morley / Diabetes / SSS-4019
	15	Martha Drake / Cough / SSS-1904
	30	
	45	
10	00	Complete — Anna Isacs / physical exam /
	15	SSS-4111
	30	↓
	45	
11	00	
	15	
	30	
	45	
12	00	Lunch
	15	
	30	
	45	
1	00	
	15	Farah Sholes / Sinuses / SSS-1918
	30	Barker Knolls / Recheck arm / SSS-1988
	45	
2	00	SSS- — Frances Dodd / Kidney infection / 1191
	15	
	30	555- — William Morgan / Remove cast / 1981
	45	
3	00	Betty Eddins / Back pain / SSS-4014
	15	
	30	Sandy Waasdorp / Checkup / SSS-9011
	45	
4	00	
	15	
	30	
	45	

WEDNESDAY July 17

9	00	
	15	
	30	
	45	
10	00	
	15	
	30	
	45	
11	00	
	15	
	30	
	45	
12	00	Lunch
	15	
	30	
	45	
1	00	
	15	
	30	
	45	
2	00	
	15	
	30	
	45	
3	00	
	15	
	30	
	45	
4	00	
	15	
	30	
	45	

Name: _____   Date: _____

Action Paper 7-8

Note from Lydia

As a review of proper scheduling procedures, I'd like you to read the scheduling instructions on our office CD and do the scheduling exercise.

Name: _____   Date: _____

To Do List

-
-
-
-
-
-
-
-
-
-
-
-
-
-
-
-

Name: _____

Date Started: _____ Date Completed: _____

Work Summary 7

Section 1

1. Record the numbers of the Action Papers marked "Rush." _____

2. Record the numbers of the Action Papers marked "ASAP." _____

3. Record the numbers of the Action Papers marked "Routine." _____

Section 2

4. Write the list of "To Do" items and the actions that were taken. When this section is complete, turn the Work Summary over to your instructor, who will evaluate your work and return it for your later use.

To Do   Action Taken

_____   _____

_____   _____

_____   _____

_____   _____

_____   _____

_____   _____

Section 3

5. You will receive two assessments for your work—one is based on time to complete the items and the other is based on quality of work. Your instructor will complete the Assessment portion of the Work Summary.

Points Received

Time Required   _____

                20 points   30 minutes or less

                15 points   40 minutes

                10 points   50 minutes

                 5 points   60 minutes

Quality of Work   _____

Total Points _____

Name: _____ Date: _____

PART III   Computers and Information Processing in the Medical Office

CHAPTER 8
Computerizing the Medical Office

Chapter Outline

Key Vocabulary Terms

Match each word or term with its correct meaning.

_____	1. Database	a.	removing an item from inventory and using it
_____	2. Graphics	b.	delay between purchase and receipt of item
_____	3. Inventory	c.	inventory items that are no longer used
_____	4. Inventory issue	d.	pictures or charts designed on a computer
_____	5. Inventory receipt	e.	calculation of rows and numbers in columns
_____	6. Lead time	f.	supplier of products or services
_____	7. Obsolete supplies	g.	creation of documents on computer, not typewriter
_____	8. PC	h.	disposing of obsolete items
_____	9. Spreadsheet	i.	personal computer
_____	10. Supply disposal	J.	software application for sorting data
_____	11. Vendor	k.	placing an item into inventory
_____	12. Word processing	l.	store of supplies

Chapter Review

1. What two factors make computers valuable to medical offices?

_____

_____

_____

_____

2. The term "computer system" refers to what components?

_____

_____

_____

_____

_____

_____

_____

_____

3. Scheduling software is an example of what basic computer function?

_____

_____

_____

_____

_____

4. For what purposes might a medical practice use graphics software?

_____

_____

_____

_____

5. For what purposes might a medical practice use desktop publishing software?

_____

_____

_____

_____

6. Drug inventories should be developed using what type of software?

_____

_____

_____

7. For what purposes might a spreadsheet be used in a medical office?

_____

_____

_____

_____

8. When would a medical assistant use presentation software?

_____

_____

_____

_____

9. Name several typical office management reports that could be developed effectively using the computer.

_____

_____

_____

_____

10. What is the key objective a medical assistant should keep in mind when purchasing supplies?

_____

_____

_____

_____

Critical Thinking Scenarios

1. Dr. Raffa tells you that she will be giving a talk at the national AMA convention in six months, and she wants to begin putting her speech together. She says, "I'll have several pages of copy and some graphs and charts. I'll have lots of lists and bulleted items to include." What type of software will provide the best solution for Dr. Raffa and why?

_____

_____

_____

_____

2. You and a Computer Salesworks representative have decided on the desktop computer that will serve you best, and the salesperson has agreed verbally to several conditions you insisted on. What follow-up steps should you take before purchasing the computer?

_____

_____

_____

_____

3. You are the office manager at a pulmonary practice that consists of five physicians, three administrative medical assistants, five clinical medical assistants, and two laboratory technologists. During the year, you spend days trying to coordinate the vacation schedule so that the office is always well covered. You are convinced that computer software will make your job simpler. What type of software would you use and what information would you include in the vacation schedule?

_____

_____

_____

_____

4. You work for a small medical practice that has difficulty keeping up with office supplies because of the poor inventory system. Copier toner and printer cartridges seem to run out at the most inconvenient times, ending with your having to go out to the office supply store in the middle of the day. How will you improve the inventory system?

_____

_____

_____

_____

5. The computer system does not malfunction too often in your office, but when it does no one seems to know how to get it up and running. Two or more days often pass before the service technician can schedule time to correct the problem. What recommendations can you make for eliminating this problem?

_____

_____

_____

_____

6. You are requested by the physician to get a brochure typeset and printed by a printing company, yet you are confident that you can design a brochure as attractive and effective using the desktop publishing software and printer in your office. What advantages might accrue from preparing the brochure in the office?

_____

_____

_____

_____

7. Long and Crecco Cardiology Associates is opening a second office and plans to invite current patients to an open house. You could use a word processing, database management, or spreadsheet program to key and print the names and addresses. Which choice will you make and why?

_____

_____

_____

_____

8. You have been asked to prepare a list of frequently used office supplies at Cortez and Lassen Medical Center. What items will you include in the list?

_____

_____

_____

_____

Simulation 8

Today is your eighth day of work at Marks and Graupera.

Supplies Needed

Blank paper
To Do List
Work Summary

Action Options, Suggestions, and Conflicts

• Use software to complete the actions in this simulation. If the software is not available, use a substitute method. For example, in Action 8-2, you may draw the business card and stationery design. In some Actions, you might substitute word processing software as the tool for completing the action.

Action Paper 8-1

Okay, this is your chance. I know you think our computer system is behind the times. Read Dr. Marks's note and tell me what activities you want a new system to handle for us — I'm interested in anything that will make your job easier.

Lydia

Marks and Graupera, P.C.

Note from Dr. Marks

Lydia, we've delayed much too long in purchasing a new computer system. Please meet with the medical assistants and develop a list of the crucial functions we want a new system to perform for the office. You and I will discuss the list, and then I'll ask you to begin calling the equipment vendors.

Action Paper 8-2

To: Your name@MarksandGraupera.com
From: LydiaMakay@MarksandGraupera.com
Subject: New business cards and stationery

I'd like to create a new design for our business cards and stationery. Will you see what you can come up with? Use a word processing program or a desktop publishing program. Here are some ideas I drafted at home last night. See whether you can come up with something more creative.

Business card
Marks and Graupera (use clip art of something medical)
Name and address
Telephone number, etc.

Stationery
Marks and Graupera   Name and address   Telephone number, etc.

Action Paper 8-3

Note from Lydia

On our office CD, you'll see samples of all the different ways we use computers. I'd like you to familiarize yourself with our computer procedures.

To Do List

-
-
-
-
-
-
-
-
-
-
-
-
-
-
-
-

Name: _____

Date Started: _____ Date Completed: _____

Work Summary 8

Section 1

1. Record the numbers of the Action Papers marked "Rush." _____

2. Record the numbers of the Action Papers marked "ASAP." _____

3. Record the numbers of the Action Papers marked "Routine." _____

Section 2

4. Write the list of "To Do" items and the actions that were taken. When this section is complete, turn the Work Summary over to your instructor, who will evaluate your work and return it for your later use.

To Do   Action Taken

_____   _____

_____   _____

_____   _____

_____   _____

_____   _____

_____   _____

Section 3

5. You will receive two assessments for your work—one is based on time to complete the items and the other is based on quality of work. Your instructor will complete the Assessment portion of the Work Summary.

Points Received

Time Required   _____

    20 points   120 minutes or less
    15 points   150 minutes
    10 points   180 minutes
     5 points   210 minutes

Quality of Work   _____

Total Points _____

CHAPTER 9
Medical Documents and Word Processing

Chapter Outline

Key Vocabulary Terms

Match each word or term with its correct meaning.

———— 1. Block

———— 2. Formatting

———— 3. Gender bias

———— 4. Gender neutral

———— 5. Modified block

———— 6. Proofread

———— 7. Redundancy

———— 8. Stored letter parts

———— 9. Thesaurus

———— 10. Tone

———— 11. Transcription

a. placement of the parts of a letter

b. to examine a document for errors

c. standard paragraphs stored in computer memory

d. to write from one source to another

e. sound of a letter

f. language that is not biased toward either sex

g. contains synonyms and antonyms

h. letter format with all lines beginning at left margin

i. unnecessary repetition of words

j. subtle form of verbal sex discrimination

k. letter format with date and closing lines at center

Chapter Review

1. What is meant by the "You" viewpoint?

_____

_____

_____

_____

2. What does "Saying 'No' in a 'Yes' way" mean?

_____

_____

_____

_____

_____

_____

_____

3. What factors should be taken into account when attempting to write at the reader's level?

_____

_____

_____

_____

_____

4. How can gender bias be eliminated in writing?

_____

_____

_____

_____

5. Why should passive voice be used infrequently in writing?

_____

_____

_____

_____

6. Why is writing a letter for the doctor's signature a challenge?

_____

_____

_____

7. What is meant by each of the following proofreader's marks?

∧ _____

[_____

] _____

=/ _____

stet _____

tr _____

// _____

lc or / _____

8. Name several sources of document input a medical assistant receives.

_____

_____

_____

_____

9. Show two methods for formatting the second page heading of a letter.

_____

_____

_____

_____

10. What is the value of merged paragraphs to a medical assistant?

_____

_____

_____

_____

Critical Thinking Scenarios

1. Sara Arker has missed her last two appointments. She will be charged for missed appointments in the future. Write a sentence or two delivering this negative message to Sara in a positive way.

_____

_____

_____

_____

2. Another staff member at Haygood and Laden has asked you to review her letter to a patient. A few sentences are reproduced below. Improve the letter.

   Mrs. Winfield, if you miss anymore appointments without calling to cancel, we will start charging you. I am sorry.

_____

_____

_____

_____

3. Sandy Fiora, another medical assistant at Manzo & Associates, P.C. says she can never think of the correct word to use when she needs it. What would you recommend to help her?

_____

_____

_____

_____

4. Because of your good writing skills, you have been chosen to help other medical assistants in the office with their writing. Help them change these passive sentences into active sentences.

The patients were impatiently waiting for the doctor to arrive.

_____

The child was crying pitifully when he was brought to the medical office.

_____

Researchers are working hard to find a cure for AIDS.

_____

The parents are working hard to provide good medical care for their children.

_____

5. Change this short, choppy sentence into a well-constructed one.

The woman was in obvious pain. She said she had a headache. Her hands were shaking.

_____

_____

_____

_____

6. As a medical office manager at Baesel and Robin, you have decided to require all medical assistants in your office to use a standard letter and punctuation format. What format will you recommend?

_____

_____

_____

_____

7. One of your friends who works as a medical assistant in another practice is worried because his employer says his letters are gender-biased. He complains that this is not a very important issue. What is your response?

_____

_____

_____

_____

8. Lately the physician has asked you to write several letters for her signature, and you are having trouble making them sound like her. What can you do about this problem?

_____

_____

_____

_____

9. You receive many rough draft documents each day to word process, and you believe you waste a great deal of time going back and forth between the rough draft and the new document. What can you do to correct the problem?

_____

_____

_____

_____

10. You have the choice of using a word processing program or a graphics program to design a brochure. Which will you use and why?

_____

_____

_____

_____

Simulation 9

Today is your ninth day of work at Marks and Graupera.

Supplies Needed

Seven sheets of blank paper
To Do List
Work Summary

Action Options, Suggestions, and Conflicts

• Key and print all documents as indicated in the instructions.

Action Paper 9-1a

Marks and Graupera, P.C.

Note from Lydia

Here is a report on telephone answering that I would like to give to all our new medical assistants. Please type this document on a word processor and print it so I can distribute it at the next staff meeting.

Good Telephone Techniques
Conducting good telephone conversations requires an understanding of basic communication skills and a desire to improve telephone techniques. Study the following techniques, then incorporate them into your daily telephone conversations.

Put Yourself in the Caller's Place
Many calls to medical offices are made by people who are sick or who are worried about a sick family member. The caller may sound impatient or irritable when this is not the case at all. In a face-to-face conversation, gestures and facial expressions give clues to the reasons for an individual's behavior. In a telephone conversation, these clues are missing. When a caller sounds unfriendly, you must use your telephone skill to determine the problem. Once you identify the problem, try to think how you would feel in a similar situation. Treat the caller as you would like to be treated.

Give Your Full Attention to the Caller
When you are talking with someone, give your full attention to that person. Answer questions fully, even though you are busy and feel rushed. Give the caller plenty of time to explain the reason for the call. Do not interrupt unless it is necessary in order to learn the reason for the call. If an emergency arises that requires you to leave the phone, tactfully explain that you must attend to an emergency and will call the person back as soon as possible. Do not ask the person to hold while you are gone.

continues

Name: _____   Date: _____

Speak Clearly and Distinctly

When you talk on the telephone, speak clearly and distinctly. Although you can hear yourself clearly, the listener may have difficulty if the mouthpiece is several inches away from your mouth. Never chew gum or eat while you talk. This noise is offensive and is distracting for the listener.

Use a Courteous Tone

Just as you are courteous when you greet a visitor to the medical office, you should also be courteous when you talk by telephone. Say "Please" and "Thank you" when appropriate. Answer the phone with a friendly greeting, such as "Good morning, Dr. Lynn's office." Close the conversation on a pleasant note, such as "Thank you, good-bye." You must make certain that outside influences do not cause you to react in a way that could be misinterpreted by the listener. Telephone courtesy should not be overlooked, even in the busy environment of a medical office.

Maintain Confidentiality

A medical secretary comes in contact with confidential information daily. This information includes medical information about patients, the personal background of patients, and personal or business facts concerning the physician or the medical office. None of this confidential information should ever be released without the physician's permission. Not only is it unethical to release confidential information, in some cases it is also illegal. For example, a person who releases medical information without a signed release statement from a patient may be sued by that patient.

Never Suggest Treatment or Medication

Since many patients see their physicians for common ailments, the medical secretary soon learns the method of treatment the physician generally prescribes. Therefore, the medical secretary might be tempted to recommend to a caller how to treat a medical problem. You must never assume that it is acceptable for you to suggest treatment. Doing so leaves both you and the physician liable for a malpractice lawsuit if a patient is physically harmed as a result of your recommendation.

Name: _____   Date: _____

Action Paper 9-2

Note from Dr. Graupera

Please improve my form letter to patients who are being referred to a specialist. I haven't liked this letter for a long time, but it always seems to go to the bottom of my stack of paperwork. Use a word processor and print your revised letter for my review.

Dear _____:

I am referring you to Dr. _____. He/She is a specialist in _____. I am sure you will like Dr. _____. I have been referring patients to him/her for many years. I have confidence in his/her ability to treat your condition. I will ask him/her to send reports to me.

I look forward to continuing to treat you for your other medical situations.

Sincerely,

Action Paper 9-3

Dr. Marks: "Lydia tells me you are an excellent letter writer. Will you draft a letter to my young cardiology patients (12 and under) inviting them to a party next month? I'm planning to bring in a ventriloquist to discuss good heart health and the things the children can do to take care of themselves. The date is 5/28, and the time is 10:30. That's a Saturday morning. We'll have treats for everyone."

You: "Of course. When do you need the letter?"

Dr. Marks: "By 2 PM today. Print a copy for me, please."

Name: _____ Date: _____

Action Paper 9-4

Please edit this letter and type it on a word processor for Dr. Graupera.

Thanks,
Lydia

May 11, 200X

Mr. Raymond R. Stogner
634 Concord Way
Wayne, PA 19087

Dear Mr. Stegner

A copy of the patient charge slip for Jason's visit on April 10 and the health insurence claim form you requested are enclosed. Please complete Items 1-12 of the claim form. Read the instructions carefully before filling in the information requested. The information you provide must be acurate and completely in order for your claim to be processed by your insurance carrier. Be sure to sign and date itemm 12.

After you have completed Items 1-12 atach the copy of the patient charge slip to the front of the form. Then mail the form (with the charge slip attached) to your insurance carrier. Please dont hesitate to contact this if you have any questions or if we can be of further help.

Sincerely

Action Paper 9-5

Here's my rough draft of Consuelo Lopez's discharge summary. I proofed it once and corrected the errors, but please proofread it again. I may have missed some. Please type in proper form and mail to the Medical Records Dept. at Metropolitan Hospital when you have time.

R.G.

Discharge Summary — Consuelo Lopez

Admitted to metropolitan Hospital: 5/ 1/——; Discharged: 5/6/——

Diagnosis at admission — Chronic urinary tract infection with renal failure. Glaucoma with resultant blindness, bilateral cataracts. Senility resulting from generalized atherosclerosis. Recent admission for acute urinary tract infection.

Discharge diagnosis — Acute renal infection, secondary to recurrent urinary tract infection.
Blindness, secondary to glaucoma; status of postoperative left cataract surgery—no improvement of vision.
Anemia, secondary to gastric irritation, hemorrhoidal bleeding, and malnourishment; recurrent infections.
Severe depression due to general weakened state.

Operations/Procedures: Removal of left cataract by Dr. Albert Iannuzzi.

INFECTION: Recurrent urinary tract infection

Condition on discharge — Poor

BRIEF HISTORY AND PHYSICAL: This 84-year-old female has a 2-year history of recurrent inflammation of the urinary bladder. She has responded well to antibiotic therapy. the day prior to admission, she complained of a frequent and urgent desire to urinate and a burning pain in the urethra during and after urination. On the day of admission, she had a temperature of 102.2 F, pain in the lumbar region, and shaking chills. There was a marked tenderness in the kidney areas. Urinalysis showed numerous white blood cells and pus. She also had a white blood count of 23,000 per cubic cm. with a shift to the left.

HOSPITAL Course: The patient was treated immediately with ampicillin since a preliminary bacterial count was in excess of 100,000 per ml. The organism was later identified as E. coli and tests showed greatest sensitivity to streptomycin. Due to impaired kidney functions, however, ampicillin therapy was continued. She was given fluids and other supportive measures. The patients condition improved markedly over the course of a few days; but due to her blindness, generalized arthritis, and weakened state, she was started on physical therapy in hopes of making her self-sufficient again. Cataract surgery was scheduled and accomplished without significant benefit. After 3 days, her urinary infection had subsided, but because of her overall weakened condition, depression, and history of infections, prognosis is not good.

DiscHARGE MEDICATIONS AND INSTRUCTIONS: Patient and family instructed to watch for symptoms of recurrent infection. Because of her weakened state, arrangements were made for patient to reside with her daughter, where the family can maintain a close watch on her condition and provide aid. She is to return to my office in two weeks for urinalysis and is to see Dr. Iannuzzi for ophthalmic follow-up in three weeks.

DISPOSITION: Home, to be seen in the office in two weeks

PROGNOSIS: Moderate

Ramon Graupera, M.D.

Action Paper 9-6

Note from Lydia

Go to our office CD and complete the Letter section of the program. It will give you a good review of letter formatting.

To Do List

-
-
-
-
-
-
-
-
-
-
-
-
-
-
-
-
-

Work Summary 9

Section 1

1. Record the numbers of the Action Papers marked "Rush." _____

2. Record the numbers of the Action Papers marked "ASAP." _____

3. Record the numbers of the Action Papers marked "Routine." _____

Section 2

4. Write the list of "To Do" items and the actions that were taken. When this section is complete, turn the Work Summary over to your instructor, who will evaluate your work and return it for your later use.

To Do   Action Taken

_____   _____

_____   _____

_____   _____

_____   _____

_____   _____

_____   _____

Section 3

5. You will receive two assessments for your work—one is based on time to complete the items and the other is based on quality of work. Your instructor will complete the Assessment portion of the Work Summary.

Points Received

Time Required   _____

            20 points   25 minutes or less
            15 points   30 minutes
            10 points   35 minutes
              5 points   40 minutes

Quality of Work   _____

Total Points _____

CHAPTER 10
Professional Activities, Travel Arrangements, and Postal and Delivery Services

Chapter Outline

Key Vocabulary Terms

Match each word or term with its correct meaning.

_____ 1. Association
_____ 2. Business class
_____ 3. Direct flight
_____ 4. Domestic mail services
_____ 5. Internet search
_____ 6. Itinerary
_____ 7. Keywords
_____ 8. Literature search
_____ 9. Non-stop
_____ 10. Objective
_____ 11. Orient

a. locating information through the Internet

b. special interests group that advocates by lobbying

c. review of published sources on specified topic

d. words that help locate information on the Internet

e. flight between two cities without plane change

f. the intent of the process

g. to provide an informational overview

h. flight between two cities without intermediate stops

i. schedule of travel

j. class that offers more amenities than coach

k. mail services performed by U.S. Postal Service

Chapter Review

1. Name some of the medical assistant's most important professional activities.

_____

_____

2. What is a search engine and how does it work?

_____

_____

_____

_____

3. List several guidelines for how patients learn best.

_____

_____

_____

_____

_____

4. Why is using the Internet an easy way to secure airline tickets?

_____

_____

_____

_____

5. What items are generally needed when the physician travels internationally?

_____

_____

_____

_____

6. What is needed to obtain a passport?

_____

_____

_____

7. Name and describe six classes of mail service.

_____

_____

_____

_____

8. Name and describe the purpose of three special mail services.

_____

_____

_____

_____

9. What is meant by underlining and annotating mail?

_____

_____

_____

_____

10. What is the recommended procedure for sorting mail?

_____

_____

_____

_____

Critical Thinking Scenarios

1. Dr. Romez asks you to locate the most current information on AIDS as soon as possible. How will you do this?

_____

_____

_____

_____

2. Another medical assistant tells you he cannot locate information about postal procedures online. What key words would you recommend he use?

_____

_____

_____

_____

3. You are having difficulty holding the attention of a group of new medical assistants you have been asked to train about the procedures used at your office. What could you do to address the problem?

_____

_____

_____

_____

4. As the receptionist at Florby and Baker Radiologists, you distribute the brochures and other literature for patients to use. You discover that patients often do not read the material. How can you encourage patients to read the material?

_____

_____

_____

_____

5. Dr. Lamberto tells you that she must be in Chicago tomorrow morning and be back by tomorrow night. She cannot leave until after 5 PM rounds tonight. She asks you to get the cheapest ticket possible right away. What procedure will you follow?

_____

_____

_____

_____

_____

6. The physician returns from an out-of-town trip and hands you airline, car, hotel, and meal receipts, directing you to "take care of them." What will you do with all of these items?

_____

_____

_____

_____

7. The physician asks you to get a patient's x-ray to a doctor in another city by the fastest way possible and to guarantee that it arrives. What postage service will you use?

_____

_____

_____

_____

8. It is long past the time that your local post office closes for the day, yet the physician has a letter he wants you to get in the mail today. What will you do?

_____

_____

_____

_____

9. By mistake you have opened a letter to Dr. Conchini that is marked "Personal" and "Confidential." You are embarrassed. What will you do?

_____

_____

_____

10. While opening the mail this morning, you discover an important legal document that requires a response. It shows a date of June 15 but today is June 23. What procedure should you follow?

_____

_____

_____

_____

Simulation 10

Today is your tenth day of work at Marks and Graupera.

Supplies Needed

Blank paper
Expense summary
To Do List
Work Summary

Action Options, Suggestions, and Conflicts

• Take action as needed.

Name: _____   Date: _____

Marks and Graupera, P.C.

Note from Dr. Marks

Suzanne Romez is busy on another project I assigned to her. Will you check some airline flights for me?

I need to be in Salt Lake City for a 3 PM meeting at one of the hospitals on a Monday in three to four weeks. The hospital there will let me choose which Monday. I would prefer to depart here on Monday morning, but I can leave on Sunday night if necessary. Please leave me at least two hours to be in Salt Lake before the meeting. I would like to take a return flight late on Monday afternoon, if possible, but be sure to get me home before 10 PM, as I want to get a good night's sleep. If I can't get into Philadelphia before 10 PM, bring me back on the first available flight on Tuesday morning.

Name: _____   Date: _____

Action Paper 10-2

Marks and Graupera, P.C.

Note from Lydia

Please go online and see what is the cheapest shipping service that will allow us to get x-rays out from our office tonight to arrive in San Francisco tomorrow by 10 AM. Try U.S. Postal Express Mail, FedEx, UPS, and, perhaps, one or two others. I don't know the Web site addresses.

Action Paper 10-3a

MEMO FROM
DR. RAMON GAUPERA

Here are my expenses for the Wellness Medicine conference I attended last week. Please organize them and develop an expense report for the accountant. Don't forget that I paid a $550 registration fee for the conference a few months ago; also, charge miles from my home to the airport and back at 36 cents a mile. It's 38 miles each direction.

Dr. G

Monday, 4/14 Limo to hotel	42.00
4/14 Monday, lunch	15.23
4/14 Taxi to convention center	11.00
Wednesday, 4/15 Taxi to convention center	11.00
Tips	12.00
4/14 Dinner with Frank Advar	158.87
4/15 Dinner with Annette Falzer	104.20
4/14–4/15 Hotel @ 178.20	356.40
Air travel from Baltimore to Cincinnati and return	347.20
Airport parking two days	28.00

Name: _____ Date: _____

Action Paper 10-3b

Travel Expense Statement

NAME _____ SOC. SEC. NO. _____

NAME _____ TRAVEL
DATES FROM _____ TO _____

PURPOSE OF TRIP _____

DATES	SPEEDOMETER READING Out / In	LOCATION/POINTS VISITED	DETAILS OF SUBSISTENCE (Attach receipts of items $25 or more)				TOTAL	Do Not Use This Space FOR ACCT. DEPT.
			BREAKFAST	LUNCH	DINNER	LODGING		

NOTE: This statement must be submitted within 10 days of last date of travel for reimbursement.

DISTANCE TRAVELLED _____ KILOMETERS @ _____ CENTS A KILOMETER
(Must be supported by automobile travel record above.)

COMMON CARRIER: _____ Taxi: _____ Limousine: _____ Airline: _____ Train: _____

MISCELLANEOUS EXPENSES: (telephone, postage, etc.):
Total here, itemize below

GRAND TOTAL OF TRAVEL EXPENSES

List all miscellaneous expenses:

Explanation _____ Amount _____

Explanation _____ Amount _____

I certify that the above statements are true and I have incurred the described expenses in the discharge of my official duties for **NORTHSIDE MEDICAL CENTER, P.C.**

SIGNATURE _____ APPROVED _____ DATE _____

Name: _____ Date: _____

To Do List

-
-
-
-
-
-
-
-
-
-
-
-
-
-
-
-

Name: _____

Date Started: _____ Date Completed: _____

Work Summary 10

Section 1

1. Record the numbers of the Action Papers marked "Rush." _____

2. Record the numbers of the Action Papers marked "ASAP." _____

3. Record the numbers of the Action Papers marked "Routine." _____

Section 2

4. Write the list of "To Do" items and the actions that were taken. When this section is complete, turn the Work Summary over to your instructor, who will evaluate your work and return it for your later use.

To Do   Action Taken

_____   _____

_____   _____

_____   _____

_____   _____

_____   _____

_____   _____

Section 3

5. You will receive two assessments for your work—one is based on time to complete the items and the other is based on quality of work. Your instructor will complete the Assessment portion of the Work Summary.

Points Received

Time Required   _____

       20 points   50 minutes or less
       15 points   60 minutes
       10 points   70 minutes
        5 points   80 minutes

Quality of Work   _____

Total Points _____

CHAPTER 11
Managing Medical Records

Chapter Outline

Key Vocabulary Terms

Match each word or term with its correct meaning.

_____ 1. Assignment of benefits

_____ 2. Blood tests

_____ 3. Capitation

_____ 4. Case history

_____ 5. Clearinghouse

_____ 6. Closed files

_____ 7. Coordination of benefits

_____ 8. Co-payment

_____ 9. Dependents

_____ 10. Disability

_____ 11. Doctor's notes

_____ 12. Electrocardiogram

_____ 13. Elimination period

_____ 14. Exclusions

_____ 15. Explanation of benefits

_____ 16. Extended benefits

_____ 17. Inactive files

_____ 18. Laboratory request

_____ 19. Pathology and cytopathology

_____ 20. Patient health questionnaire

_____ 21. Patient information form

_____ 22. Problem-oriented medical record

_____ 23. Shingling

_____ 24. SOAP

_____ 25. Source-oriented medical record

_____ 26. Urinalysis

_____ 27. X-rays, CAT scans, and ultrasound

a. records of patients not seen in some time

b. questions about a patient's medical history

c. reporting of diagnoses and treatments

d. benefits signed over from an insurance payment to a third party

e. doctor comments added to medical record

f. method of filing small reports

g. amount policyholder pays for each visit

h. services not paid by insurance

i. report detailing reimbursement

j. time between disability and start of benefits

k. form completed by patient for the first visit

l. pay based on number of policy members

m. information grouped according to source

n. medical records of past patients

o. patient's complaints in list form

p. routine laboratory test of urine

q. tests used to determine unusual conditions

r. graphic illustration of the heart's activity

s. central claims distribution center

t. comprehensive patient history

u. laboratory testing of body tissue and body cells

v. financial responsibility limitation clause

w. wife and children of insurance policyholder

x. injury or illness that affects ability to work

y. supplemental coverage to a basic plan

z. type of test requested and name of physician

aa. analysis of blood

Chapter Review

1. What is a medical record?

_____

_____

_____

_____

2. Why must medical records be complete and accurate?

_____

_____

_____

_____

3. List several methods that are used for keeping medical records.

_____

_____

_____

_____

_____

4. What is the concept behind color coding of medical records?

_____

_____

_____

_____

5. Name some of the items contained in a medical record.

_____

_____

_____

_____

6. What is a problem-oriented medical record?

_____

_____

_____

_____

7. What is a source-oriented medical record?

_____

_____

_____

_____

8. What are active files and what are closed files?

_____

_____

_____

_____

9. Why is numeric filing used instead of alphabetic filing in some medical offices?

_____

_____

_____

_____

10. When would subject files be used in a medical office?

_____

_____

_____

_____

Critical Thinking Scenarios

1. In passing by the files, you notice that a folder with a brown label is mixed in with the blue-labeled folders. What is the problem and how will you correct it?

_____

_____

_____

_____

2. When you empty your in-basket, you come upon a loose laboratory report for a patient whose name you do not recognize. What will you do with it and why?

_____

_____

_____

_____

3. Currently, all patients who have not seen the physician for five years have their folders in one location. The file cabinets are bulging and you know you have to reduce the number of folders in some way. What storage procedure changes might you recommend?

_____

_____

_____

_____

4. Dr. Renisky is often rushed, and sometimes you are concerned that he forgets to dictate a follow-up after seeing patients in the hospital or nursing home. What can you do to ensure that all folders have up-to-date information?

_____

_____

_____

_____

5. Most of Dr. Mulmory's correspondence that is unrelated to patients has to do with his research into dermatological problems. Currently, these documents are all stored in several files labeled "Dermatology research." How could you improve on this method?

_____

_____

_____

_____

_____

6. Records with the following patients' names are in a tray for filing. In what order should you arrange the names for correct alphabetic filing?

Raymond Van Cleef, Solomon Vance, Royce Vancleef, Abby Van, Veronica Van Cleef

_____

_____

_____

_____

7. Many of the laboratory reports received in your office come on small or odd-sized pieces of paper. What method of filing do you recommend for efficiency?

_____

_____

_____

_____

8. Folders with the following tabs appear in your subject files. In what order should they be stored?

AAA, Triple A Uniforms, AAA Movers, A A A Laboratory Supplies

_____

_____

_____

_____

9. A new patient by the name of Sanella Di Pre has recently seen the doctor. She also goes by the name Mrs. Jacque Di Pre. You are concerned that you will be unable to locate her folder. How can you guard against this?

_____

_____

_____

10. In the rush to get her work done each day, you notice that one of the medical assistants in your office hurriedly places patient information in the medical records. On a few occasions, you have found medical records out of order, and she has apologized by saying, "Sorry, I was in a hurry." What advice do you have for this medical assistant?

_____

_____

_____

_____

Simulation 11

Today is your eleventh day of work at Marks and Graupera.

Supplies Needed

Two sheets of blank paper
To Do List
Work Summary

Action Options, Suggestions, and Conflicts

- When filing the Action Papers for training days 1–15, discard any that would not normally be filed.

Action Paper 11-1

To: Your name@MarksandGraupera.com
From: LydiaMakay@aol.com
Subject: File folder label

Please set up the file folder tabs for Elisha Tandy's medical record. She was last here in 2004.

Action Paper 11-2

Marks and Graupera, P.C.

Note from Lydia

Several new patients are expected this week, and we're also establishing relationships with a number of new suppliers. Will you please get a head start by preparing a list of the file folder labels we will need? Index the names, then make a list of all the labels in correct alphabetic filing order. For the nonpatient files, use the tabs you established before and add new ones if needed. Thanks for your help.

Rev. Du Pont, patient
Samuel Arthur Clark, patient
Harris of Philadelphia Laboratory Supplies
John Martin Pediatrics
Lowen Raycheck, patient
Martin Prosthetics Company
Arthur Sylvester, patient
Dr. Ester Diaz
MacDonald Druggists
Metro Ambulance Service, 1802 Reynolds Lane
Lewis Raychen, patient
Arthur Sylvester, Sr., patient
Carla Walgreen, M.D.
Mrs. Nobel D. Brown (Fay Brown), patient
Clark Printing
Valerie Wiley Flower Shop
Ai-ling Cheng
The Wm. A. Williams Corporation
Metropolitan Ambulance Service, 2045 Peyton Lane
Donna Di George, patient
Dr. Sarah Jane Du Pont
Arthur Sylvester, Jr., patient
Walter Armstrong-Jones, patient
Williams Uniforms
Fiona Browne, patient
Mrs. Carl Henry Sanders (Mrs. Ellen Theresa Sanders), patient
Sra Ling Pei
McDonald Drugs
Sara Ling
A-1 Orthopedic Supplies
Opti-Care Center
Wm. A. Wms & Sons
Sera Pei

Name: _____   Date: _____

Action Paper 11-3

Tarik: "Hi (your name). Lydia told me she gave you some new filing projects. Our office CD has really good information on filing and some filing exercises to give you practice. There's also a section on tickler files. I recommend you go through all the filing suggestions on the CD before you start the work Lydia gave you."

Name: _____   Date: _____

To Do List

-
-
-
-
-
-
-
-
-
-
-
-
-
-
-
-

Name: _____

Date Started: _____ Date Completed: _____

Work Summary 11

Section 1

1. Record the numbers of the Action Papers marked "Rush."   _____

2. Record the numbers of the Action Papers marked "ASAP."   _____

3. Record the numbers of the Action Papers marked "Routine." _____

Section 2

4. Write the list of "To Do" items and the actions that were taken. When this section is complete, turn the Work Summary over to your instructor, who will evaluate your work and return it for your later use.

To Do   Action Taken

_____   _____

_____   _____

_____   _____

_____   _____

_____   _____

_____   _____

Section 3

5. You will receive two assessments for your work—one is based on time to complete the items and the other is based on quality of work. Your instructor will complete the Assessment portion of the Work Summary.

                                                              Points Received

Time Required   _____

    20 points   80 minutes or less
    15 points   90 minutes
    10 points   100 minutes
     5 points   110 minutes

Quality of Work   _____

                              Total Points _____

PART IV   Automating Medical Office Financial Management

CHAPTER 12
Pegboard Accounting and Computerized Account Management

Chapter Outline

Key Vocabulary Terms

Match each word or term with its correct meaning.

_____ 1. Balance

_____ 2. Charge slip

_____ 3. *CPT*

_____ 4. Daily log

_____ 5. Electronic fund transfer

_____ 6. FICA

_____ 7. Form W-2

_____ 8. Form W-4

_____ 9. ICD codes

_____ 10. Ledger card

_____ 11. Overdraft

_____ 12. Pegboard accounting

_____ 13. Practice analysis

_____ 14. Proof of posting

_____ 15. Reconciliation

a. verification of practice account balances and bank account balances

b. a check that exceeds the bank balance

c. a form that lists an employee's taxation exemptions

d. receipt listing treatments, services, or procedures

e. overview of procedures and treatments provided

f. a method of maintaining accounts

g. verification of daily log calculations

h. the day's summary of patient transactions

i. moving money through a computer network

j. amount in a checking account at any time

k. annual form that summarizes an employee's earnings, deductions, and net income

l. the act that set up Social Security funding

m. diagnosis codes

n. the record of checking account information

o. treatment, services, and procedure codes

Chapter Review

1. Name and describe the three components of a pegboard accounting system.

_____

_____

_____

_____

2. ICD is short for what term? For what purpose is ICD used?

_____

_____

_____

_____

3. What procedure should be followed when receiving checks?

_____

_____

_____

_____

_____

4. Explain the process of reconciliation of a bank statement.

_____

_____

_____

_____

5. Describe the four electronic banking systems that a medical office assistant may use.

_____

_____

_____

6. Explain the role of Form W-4 in an employee's taxes.

_____

_____

_____

7. What information is provided on a daily list of appointments?

_____

_____

_____

_____

8. What is the purpose of an employee earnings record?

_____

_____

_____

_____

9. What type of tax is FICA and for what reason are FICA taxes collected?

_____

_____

_____

_____

10. Compare and contrast a pegboard accounting system and a computerized accounting system.

_____

_____

_____

Critical Thinking Scenarios

1. An argumentative patient tells you that she does not owe a bill because she has not been to the office in the past six months. What document will you locate to identify when the patient was in the office last?

_____

2. Dr. Roswell wants to compare the practice's financial activities for the past three Fridays. What document will you locate to provide this information?

_____

3. You have written a $75 check to replenish petty cash. On which financial document will you make a note about this check?

_____

4. You are training a newly hired collection clerk and are explaining why controlling accounts receivable is so important. What do you tell her?

_____

_____

_____

_____

5. As you walk by the accounts payable clerk's desk, you notice that he writes several checks, then he goes back and fills in the check stub. As his supervisor, what recommendations should you make to him?

_____

_____

_____

6. Bank reconciliation takes a good deal of time, and you are wondering whether you might be able to give up this responsibility. What are the reasons for continuing?

_____

_____

_____

7. On what occasions might you want to recommend to the physicians that they move money from one account to another by electronic transfer?

_____

_____

_____

_____

8. One of the medical assistants asks you how many exemptions she can claim. She is unmarried. What is your answer?

_____

_____

_____

_____

9. Another medical assistant has two children and an ex-husband. She wonders how many exemptions she can claim. What is your answer?

_____

_____

_____

10. A new employee wants to deduct "as little as possible" from her paycheck. She asks you what deductions are required. What is your answer?

_____

_____

Simulation 12

Today is your twelfth day of work at Marks and Graupera.

Supplies Needed

Blank check
Daily log
Health Insurance Claim Form
To Do List
Work Summary

Action Options, Suggestions, and Conflicts

• Use the Reference Sheet to help you complete the Action Papers.

Name: _____   Date: _____

Note from Lydia

Please finalize the patient charge slips for five patients. Show the diagnosis and diagnosis codes, mark the CPT codes, list the fees, and write any instructions for the patient given by Dr. Graupera.

Arash Bonaker, Account No. 615, of 201 Tanglewood Court, Wayne, PA 19087, telephone number 610-555-9876, was in today for treatment of potential hepatitis. Mr. Bonaker is a security officer at Valley Forge National Park. His insurer is Metropolitan Medical Insurers, and his policy number is MIC –4326B. His group plan number is VFNP 101. There are no other insurers. His date of birth is 6/6/63.

He had an intermediate office visit, a CBC, and a hematocrit. His primary symptoms are malaise and headaches. He has five old tattoos on his upper torso and arms, which suggest hepatitis. He should return in five days for follow-up and testing for Lyme disease.

He may continue working as long as he feels well enough. His wife will call in two days with an update on his progress.

He wants to pay his bill in full, including his previous balance.

PATIENT CHARGE SLIP
Marks and Graupera, P.C.
2201 Locust Street
Philadelphia, PA 19101
215-283-8372

DATE	PATIENT	SERVICES	CHARGE	PAYMENT	CURRENT BALANCE	PREVIOUS BALANCE	ACCOUNT NO.
	Bonaker					80.00	

Office Care	CPT	Hypothetical Fee
Brief Service	90040	_____
Limited Service	90050	_____
Intermediate Service	90060	_____
Extended Service	90070	_____
Comprehensive Service		
Established Patient	90080	_____
New Patient		
Complete Exam	90020	_____
Emergency—Acute Illness	99058	_____
Emergency After Hours	90050	_____

Office Procedures and Laboratory Work	CPT	Hypothetical Fee
Injection		
Type _____	_____	_____
Urinalysis	81000	_____
Hematocrit	85014	_____
Complete Blood Count	85022	_____
Throat Culture	87060	_____
Hepatitis C-AB	86803	_____
T4, Total	84436	_____
Triglycerides	84478	_____
Other	_____	_____

Hospital Care		
Limited Service	90285	_____
Extended Service	90270	_____
Comprehensive Service	90280	_____
Emergency Room	99062	_____

Symptoms: _____

Diagnosis: _____

Instructions: _____

Return: _____ Days _____ Weeks _____ Months

Action Paper 12-2

Andrea Swazer, Account No. 715, of 120-B King Road, Apartment 23, Malvern, PA 19355, telephone number 610-555-3829, saw Dr. Graupera for wheezing and coughing. She is an office manager at Twinkle Products, and her insurer is Banner Medical Plan, Policy No. BMP 1292, Group No. 23-B23. Her husband, Eric Swazer, of the same address, is self-employed at Swazer Deli and is insured by Philadelphia Mutual Corporation, Policy No. 574930286, Group No. XC398. His birth date is 7/3/51.

Mrs. Swazer was born on 3/30/46. Dr. Graupera diagnosed acute bronchitis. Mrs. Swazer had an intermediate office visit, a urinalysis, and a CBC. Dr. Graupera wrote her a prescription for a chest x-ray at Center City Hospital. She should have three days of bed rest. She is paying $40 of her bill.

PATIENT CHARGE SLIP
Marks and Graupera, P.C.
2201 Locust Street
Philadelphia, PA 19101
215-283-8372

DATE	PATIENT	SERVICES	CHARGE	PAYMENT	CURRENT BALANCE	PREVIOUS BALANCE	ACCOUNT NO.
	Swazer					0.00	

Office Care	CPT	Hypothetical Fee
Brief Service	90040	_____
Limited Service	90050	_____
Intermediate Service	90060	_____
Extended Service	90070	_____
Comprehensive Service		
Established Patient	90080	_____
New Patient		
Complete Exam	90020	_____
Emergency—Acute Illness	99058	_____
Emergency After Hours	90050	_____

Office Procedures and Laboratory Work	CPT	Hypothetical Fee
Injection		
Type _____	_____	_____
Urinalysis	81000	_____
Hematocrit	85014	_____
Complete Blood Count	85022	_____
Throat Culture	87060	_____
Hepatitis C-AB	86803	_____
T4, Total	84436	_____
Triglycerides	84478	_____
Other	_____	_____

Hospital Care	CPT	Hypothetical Fee
Limited Service	90285	_____
Extended Service	90270	_____
Comprehensive Service	90280	_____
Emergency Room	99062	_____

Symptoms: _____

Diagnosis: _____

Instructions: _____

Return: _____ Days _____ Weeks _____ Months

Action Paper 12-3

Sandra Hight, Account No. 412. Her birth date is 3/14/48. Mrs. Hight lives at 976 Baron Lane, Paoli, PA 19301, telephone number 610-555-2837. She saw Dr. Graupera for chest pain. Her diagnosis is chest pain, unspecified. Her husband, George, has insurance with National HMO, Policy No. 365-893XT, and his group number is Laflin RP. He is employed by Laflin Communications Service. His birth date is 6/16/41.

She had an extended office visit and an EKG. Dr. Graupera wrote a prescription for a coronary risk profile at Center City Hospital. She is to return in two weeks for follow-up. She will pay $75 today.

PATIENT CHARGE SLIP
Marks and Graupera, P.C.
2201 Locust Street
Philadelphia, PA 19101
215-283-8372

DATE	PATIENT	SERVICES	CHARGE	PAYMENT	CURRENT BALANCE	PREVIOUS BALANCE	ACCOUNT NO.
	Hight					0.00	

Office Care	CPT	Hypothetical Fee
Brief Service	90040	_____
Limited Service	90050	_____
Intermediate Service	90060	_____
Extended Service	90070	_____
Comprehensive Service		
Established Patient	90080	_____
New Patient		
Complete Exam	90020	_____
Emergency—Acute Illness	99058	_____
Emergency After Hours	90050	_____

Office Procedures and Laboratory Work	CPT	Hypothetical Fee
Injection		
Type _____		_____
Urinalysis	81000	_____
Hematocrit	85014	_____
Complete Blood Count	85022	_____
Throat Culture	87060	_____
Hepatitis C-AB	86803	_____
T4, Total	84436	_____
Triglycerides	84478	_____
Other	_____	_____

Hospital Care	CPT	Hypothetical Fee
Limited Service	90285	_____
Extended Service	90270	_____
Comprehensive Service	90280	_____
Emergency Room	99062	_____

Symptoms: _____

Diagnosis: _____

Instructions: _____

Return: _____ Days _____ Weeks _____ Months

Action Paper 12-4

Cynthia Rambo, Account No. 352, of 2304 Devon Road, Lebanon, TN 37087, telephone number 615-555-8729. Miss Rambo, who is visiting her aunt, is nauseous and is experiencing several stomach pain. She is to return in three days if her condition has not improved.

Miss Rambo's father, Stabrook Rambo, is the insured and lives at the same address. His plan is with Nashville Universal Plan, No. 3876, Group No. ABAB. He is employed by the Opryland Hotel, and his birth date is 9/27/65.

Miss Rambo had an extended office visit and a urinalysis. Dr. Graupera is referring her to Metropolitan Hospital for an abdomen survey and an upper GI. He diagnosed abdominal pain, unspecific, and abdominal swelling.

The patient's birth date is February 3, 1975. She is a full-time student. Her aunt wants to make full payment.

PATIENT CHARGE SLIP
Marks and Graupera, P.C.
2201 Locust Street
Philadelphia, PA 19101
215-283-8372

DATE	PATIENT	SERVICES	CHARGE	PAYMENT	CURRENT BALANCE	PREVIOUS BALANCE	ACCOUNT NO.
_____	Rambo	_____	_____	_____	_____	0.00	_____

Office Care	CPT	Hypothetical Fee
Brief Service	90040	_____
Limited Service	90050	_____
Intermediate Service	90060	_____
Extended Service	90070	_____
Comprehensive Service		
Established Patient	90080	_____
New Patient		
Complete Exam	90020	_____
Emergency—Acute Illness	99058	_____
Emergency After Hours	90050	_____

Office Procedures and Laboratory Work	CPT	Hypothetical Fee
Injection		
Type _____	_____	_____
Urinalysis	81000	_____
Hematocrit	85014	_____
Complete Blood Count	85022	_____
Throat Culture	87060	_____
Hepatitis C-AB	86803	_____
T4, Total	84436	_____
Triglycerides	84478	_____
Other	_____	_____

Hospital Care	CPT	Hypothetical Fee
Limited Service	90285	_____
Extended Service	90270	_____
Comprehensive Service	90280	_____
Emergency Room	99062	_____

Symptoms: _____

_____

Diagnosis: _____

Instructions: _____

Return: _____ Days _____ Weeks _____ Months

Name: _____   Date: _____

Margaret Stryker is one of Dr. Graupera's patients who has multiple sclerosis and comes in every three months for a routine checkup. Dr. Graupera has referred her to Center City Hospital for an MRI Head. Her account number is 297, and her address is 2973 Lancaster Avenue East, Strafford, PA 19087, telephone number 610-555-9276. Dr. Graupera will call her after he receives her lab reports, and she is to return in six months.

Margaret's insurance is United Health Care, Plan No. 8267, Group No. BN87-9. She is employed by the National Constitution Center, and her birth date is May 17, 1976. She had an intermediate office visit. She is also insured under her husband, Jose's, policy with Metropolitan Medical Insurance, No. MIC- 8376H. He works at the National Academy of Music and was born on January 1, 1975. She is paying $90.

PATIENT CHARGE SLIP
Marks and Graupera, P.C.
2201 Locust Street
Philadelphia, PA 19101
215-283-8372

DATE	PATIENT	SERVICES	CHARGE	PAYMENT	CURRENT BALANCE	PREVIOUS BALANCE	ACCOUNT NO.
	Stryker					182.00	

Office Care	CPT	Hypothetical Fee
Brief Service	90040	_____
Limited Service	90050	_____
Intermediate Service	90060	_____
Extended Service	90070	_____
Comprehensive Service		
Established Patient	90080	_____
New Patient		
Complete Exam	90020	_____
Emergency—Acute Illness	99058	_____
Emergency After Hours	90050	_____

Office Procedures and Laboratory Work	CPT	Hypothetical Fee
Injection		
Type _____	_____	_____
Urinalysis	81000	_____
Hematocrit	85014	_____
Complete Blood Count	85022	_____
Throat Culture	87060	_____
Hepatitis C-AB	86803	_____
T4, Total	84436	_____
Triglycerides	84478	_____
Other	_____	_____

Hospital Care	CPT	Hypothetical Fee
Limited Service	90285	_____
Extended Service	90270	_____
Comprehensive Service	90280	_____
Emergency Room	99062	_____

Symptoms: _____

Diagnosis: _____

Instructions: _____

Return: _____ Days _____ Weeks _____ Months

Please write a check for Dr. Marks' signature.
Lydia

INVOICE

To: Marks & Graupera, P.C.
From: American Uniform Company
2002 Ardith Way
Wayne, PA 19087

22 Smocks @14.92	328.24
40 gowns @ 4.09	163.60
50 tissue slippers @ 1.92	96.00
Subtotal:	491.85
Tax:	16.37
Total:	508.22

Past Due

Action Paper 12-7

Note from Lydia

Please go to the insurance section of our office CD and complete all the exercises related to insurance and coding. Use the case files on the desk as resource documents to your work.

Reference Sheet for Action Papers 12-1 through 12-5

Dr. Graupera's Fees

Office Care

Brief Service	$ 50
Limited Service	$ 60
Intermediate Service	$ 70
Extended Service	$ 80
Comprehensive Service	$125
Established Patient	
New Patient	
Complete Exam	$125
Emergency—Acute Illness	$ 80
Emergency After Hours	$225
Telephone Consultation	$ 50

Hospital Care

Limited Service	$ 80
Extended Service	$125
Comprehensive Service	$175
Emergency Room	$225

Office Procedures and Laboratory Work

Injection	$ 14
Suture	$ 8
Urinalysis	$ 8
Hematocrit	$ 43
Complete Blood Count	$ 32
Throat Culture	$ 12
PAP Smear	$ 65
Hepatitis C-AB	$ 42
T4	$ 25
Triglycerides	$ 20

ICD Codes

Abdominal pain, unspecified site	789.00
Abdominal swelling	789.30
Abnormal EKG	794.31
Abnormal heart sounds	785.3
Acute bronchitis	466.0
Anemia, iron deficiency	281.0
Angina pectoris	413.9
Aortic valve disorder	424.1
Achilles tendon tear	845.09
Acne	706.1
Abnormal liver	794
Cardiovascular disease	v17.4
Congestive heart failure	428.0
Contusion	924.9
Convulsions, other	780.39
Coronary atherosclerosis	414.01, 414.00
Coronary insufficiency	411.8
Cough	786.2
Cramps, lower extremities	729.82
Foreign body, swallowed	938
Frequent urination	788.42
Fungus infection	117.9
Gallbladder disease	575.9
Gallstones	574.2
Gas pain	787.3
Gastritis	535.0
Gastroenteritis and colitis	558.9
General medical exam	780.9
Goiter	240.9
Gout	274.9
Graves disease	240.9
Headache	784.0
Heart disease, unspecified	429.9
Hepatitis, unspecified	573.3
Hypertension, essential, benign	301.1
Hypothyroidism, unspecified	244.9
Infant or child health check, routine	v20.2
Ischemic heart disease, chronic	414.9
Kidney and ureter disorder, unspecified	593.9
Long term current use of medications	v58.69
Multiple sclerosis	340
Palpitations	785.1
Pneumonia, organism unspecified	486
Postmenopausal atrophic vaginitis	627.3
Thyroid disorder, unspecified	246.9
Tonsilitis, acute	463
Urinary frequency	788.41
Weight gain, abnormal	783.1
Weight loss, abnormal	783.2

Name: _____ Date: _____

To Do List

-

-

-

-

-

-

-

-

-

-

-

-

-

-

-

-

Name: _____

Date Started: _____ Date Completed: _____

Work Summary 12

Section 1

1. Record the numbers of the Action Papers marked "Rush." _____

2. Record the numbers of the Action Papers marked "ASAP." _____

3. Record the numbers of the Action Papers marked "Routine." _____

Section 2

4. Write the list of "To Do" items and the actions that were taken. When this section is complete, turn the Work Summary over to your instructor, who will evaluate your work and return it for your later use.

To Do   Action Taken

_____   _____

_____   _____

_____   _____

_____   _____

_____   _____

_____   _____

Section 3

5. You will receive two assessments for your work—one is based on time to complete the items and the other is based on quality of work. Your instructor will complete the Assessment portion of the Work Summary.

                                                                Points Received

Time Required   _____
                    20 points   50 minutes or less
                    15 points   60 minutes
                    10 points   70 minutes
                     5 points   80 minutes

Quality of Work   _____

                                    Total Points _____

CHAPTER 13
Billing and Collection

Chapter Outline

Billing Patients
    Internal Billing
        Charge Slip as Statement at Time of Service
        Billing Statement
        Ledger Card as Statement
        Special Statement Form
        Computerized Statement
    Monthly Billing and Cycle Billing
        Monthly Billing
        Cycle Billing
    External Billing Service
The Collection Process
    Aging Accounts
    Collection Letters Series
        Collection Letters to Patients
        Collection Letters to Third-Party Carriers
    Telephone Collections
Truth-in-Lending
Chapter Activities
    Performance-Based Activities
    Expanding Your Thinking

Key Vocabulary Terms

Match each word or term with its correct meaning.

_____ 1. Cycle billing

_____ 2. Third-party payers

_____ 3. Receivables

_____ 4. Balance

_____ 5. Billing

_____ 6. Account aging

_____ 7. Invoice

_____ 8. Payables

_____ 9. Collection

a. amount remaining owed

b. method for reporting how long an account is overdue

c. reminding patients that an amount is owed

d. others who pay the patient's bill

e. amount owed to a practice

f. statement of services

g. process for expediting overdue accounts

h. spreading billing over several days

i. amount owed by a practice

Chapter Review

1. What is the medical assistant's role in billing patients?

_____

_____

_____

_____

2. What are the advantages and disadvantages of internal billing?

_____

_____

_____

_____

3. When is the best time to collect a bill and why is this a good time?

_____

_____

_____

_____

4. What is the advantage of computerized billing of patient accounts?

_____

_____

_____

_____

5. What is the primary determining factor in whether a practice uses monthly billing or cycle billing for sending statements to patients?

_____

_____

_____

_____

6. What are the advantages and disadvantages of monthly billing and cycle billing?

_____

_____

_____

_____

7. What does the term "account aging" mean?

_____

_____

_____

_____

8. At what point should telephone collection procedures begin?

_____

_____

_____

_____

9. List several dos and don'ts for telephone collection.

_____

_____

_____

_____

10. What is the purpose of the Truth-in-Lending Act?

_____

_____

_____

_____

Critical Thinking Scenarios

1. As medical office manager, you are having difficulty getting the receptionist to accept his responsibility to ask patients for payment when they check out. He says he does not want the patients to think he is badgering them for money. Below write the comment you would like him to make to the patients as they stop by his desk to obtain their patient charge slip.

_____

_____

_____

_____

2. Monahan and Norway Pulmonary Associates has always used monthly billing; however, due to the growth of the practice, you believe that cycle billing would be more efficient. You plan to talk with Dr. Monahan and Dr. Norway about changing. What points will you make?

_____

_____

_____

_____

3. The billing clerk at Snyder OB/GYN Associates tells you that some patients tend to ignore his collection letters after their baby is born. He believes the practice needs to do something stronger to collect payment. As office manager, what is the next step you would recommend?

_____

_____

_____

_____

4. Eloise, a bright young billing clerk who has been at the job for three weeks, cannot understand why the practice ages Medicare patients' accounting differently. She says, "We give Medicare patients a bigger break on paying." She believes that Medicare patients should have to pay "on time" just like everyone else. What do you tell her?

_____

_____

_____

_____

5. As a new employee at Grandis and Vakergard, a practice that does not conduct computerized aging, you believe the practice's method of identifying overdue balances is very complicated. You decide to suggest a very simple paper method for recognizing overdue accounts. What will you recommend?

_____

_____

_____

_____

6. As an office manager at Reilley and Obrien, you are considering the use of an external billing service. The doctors ask what services an external billing service offers and how this might be helpful to the practice. What will you tell them?

_____

_____

_____

_____

_____

7. Having recently been hired to handle billing at the practice of Blackwell and Smart P.C., you believe their aging system is archaic and you hope to be able to increase efficiency with a new system. What standard aging system will you recommend?

_____

_____

_____

_____

8. The physicians at Chairwell and Stainway have decided to accept accounts on credit, and you are asked to find out what is required under the Consumer Credit Protection Act. What will you tell the physicians?

_____

_____

_____

_____

9. You decide to provide training to the collection clerk at your medical practice. What pointers will you give him?

_____

_____

_____

_____

10. You overhear the following conversation between the collection clerk and a patient. What mistakes did the clerk make?

Collection clerk: *I understand that your husband is out of work, but that's not our problem. We need our money.*

Patient: ―――――

Collection clerk: *No, I don't want to listen any longer; you're just making excuses.*

Patient: ―――――

Collection clerk: *No, you can't talk to the doctor. He is busy with another patient. If you weren't satisfied with your treatment, you should have called sooner. It's too late now.*

Patient: ―――――

Collection clerk: *Well, I don't like your attitude either. We're going to turn your account over to a collector.*

_____

_____

_____

_____

Simulation 13

Today is your thirteenth day of work at Marks and Graupera.

Supplies Needed

Six sheets of blank paper
To Do List
Work Summary

Action Options, Suggestions, and Conflicts

• Complete the Action Papers as directed or according to your judgment.

Action Paper 13-1

I'm impressed with the memos and e-mails you've written. Will you write a rough draft series of collection letters for us? Print a copy of each for our review. Thanks.

Lydia

Note from Dr. Marks

Lydia, at a meeting last night, some of the physicians were discussing that their collection letters need to be more strongly worded. Will you ask one of the medical assistants to draft us a new series for your review? Then I'd like to discuss the letters with you. We don't want to offend our patients, but we do need to collect from them.

Action Paper 13-2

E-mail from Lydia

I am going to hire an outside firm to do telephone collections for us in cases where your collection letter series doesn't get payment. Will you write a script I can give the callers to use? Assume that this is the first phone call that patients have gotten since they received the collection letter series.

Name: _____   Date: _____

Tarik: "I heard you're ready to get into billing and collections. Big job! Here's a hint. Go to the Billing and Collection section of the office CD and complete the exercises before you do anything else. There are sections called Patient Fees, Daily Log, and Receipt—all are helpful."

You: "Great, thanks."

To Do List

-
-
-
-
-
-
-
-
-
-
-
-
-
-
-
-
-

Name: _____

Date Started: _____ Date Completed: _____

Work Summary 13

Section 1

1. Record the numbers of the Action Papers marked "Rush." _____

2. Record the numbers of the Action Papers marked "ASAP." _____

3. Record the numbers of the Action Papers marked "Routine." _____

Section 2

4. Write the list of "To Do" items and the actions that were taken. When this section is complete, turn the Work Summary over to your instructor, who will evaluate your work and return it for your later use.

To Do   Action Taken

_____   _____

_____   _____

_____   _____

_____   _____

_____   _____

_____   _____

Section 3

5. You will receive two assessments for your work—one is based on time to complete the items and the other is based on quality of work. Your instructor will complete the Assessment portion of the Work Summary.

                                                                    Points Received

Time Required   _____
              20 points   75 minutes or less
              15 points   80 minutes
              10 points   85 minutes
               5 points   90 minutes

Quality of Work   _____

                                        Total Points _____

CHAPTER 14
Health Insurance and Coding

Chapter Outline

Key Vocabulary Terms

Match each word or term with its correct meaning.

_____ 1. Basic insurance

_____ 2. Commercial insurance

_____ 3. Waiver

_____ 4. Exclusion

_____ 5. Coordination of benefits

_____ 6. Waiting period

_____ 7. Major medical insurance

_____ 8. Medicaid

_____ 9. Comprehensive insurance

_____ 10. Usual and customary care

_____ 11. DRG

_____ 12. Deductible

_____ 13. Co-payment

_____ 14. Blue Cross and Blue Shield

_____ 15. Claim form

_____ 16. Prospective payment

_____ 17. Capitation

_____ 18. Worker's compensation insurance

a. amount of payment for which patient is responsible

b. amount paid by patient prior to the beginning of insurance benefits

c. method of classifying patient into categories based on the primary diagnosis

d. sharing the cost of treatment by several insurance companies

e. a fee that is usually charged for a service in a specific geographic area

f. illnesses or injuries not covered under an insurance policy

g. government insurance that protects the poor

h. documentation required by an insurance company before a claim will be paid

i. benefits that cover physicians' fees, hospital expenses, and surgical fees as determined by the contract plan

j. time between when an insurance policy is approved and the patient is covered for benefits

k. for-profit companies offering health insurance

l. combination of basic and major medical insurance

m. a policy attachment that excludes specific preexisting conditions

n. nonprofit insurers that pay for physicians' services and hospital costs

o. a method of flat fee pricing

p. employer-paid insurance that provides health care and income to employees and their dependents when employees suffer work-related injuries

q. a physician is paid a certain amount per patient

Chapter Review

1. How does basic insurance differ from major medical insurance?

_____

_____

_____

_____

2. What is the difference between traditional insurance and managed care?

_____

_____

_____

_____

3. To what does "usual and customary fee" refer?

_____

_____

_____

_____

_____

4. Explain the concept of a health maintenance organization.

_____

_____

_____

_____

5. Name and describe two types of coverage in a managed care system.

_____

_____

_____

_____

6. Which citizens does Medicare cover?

_____

_____

_____

7. What are diagnosis-related groups and how do they work?

_____

_____

_____

_____

8. What is the purpose of the Health Insurance Portability and Accounting Act?

_____

_____

_____

_____

9. Describe the route an insurance form takes from start to finish.

_____

_____

_____

_____

10. What is an audit trail and what is its purpose?

_____

_____

_____

Critical Thinking Scenarios

1. A young patient in the internal medicine practice where you work tells you that he is about to go off his parents' medical policy because he will soon be graduating. He asks you what coverage he needs to be "fully insured" in his new career as a race car driver. What will you tell him?

_____

_____

_____

_____

2. An elderly patient tells you she cannot understand why her doctors' visits are so expensive. She tells you she has the best insurance you can get—the "traditional" type she says—but she is upset because her neighbor pays only $5 for an office visit. She cannot understand why she has to pay so much more. What will you tell her?

_____

_____

_____

_____

3. When a patient calls to schedule an appointment at Lambert and Gayle Rheumatology and you ask what type of insurance coverage he has, he tells you he is covered by a PPO. You ask who the referring physician is, and he says he does not have one—that he is allowed to self-refer for an additional fee. You suggest another type of coverage and ask whether that coverage is what he has. He answers, "Yes." What coverage did you suggest?

_____

_____

_____

_____

4. A patient asks whether she can talk to you about the new insurance she is thinking about purchasing. She is concerned that it will not cover her visits to your office. Unfortunately, the patient cannot clearly describe the plan she is interested in. She tells you that it sounds like it has something to do with food. Make a suggestion as to the type of plan she may be considering. Give her a few clues that will help her decide whether this is the plan she wants to discuss. Do you have any advice for the patient?

_____

_____

_____

_____

5. A new medical assistant at the physical therapy office where you work is confused because many of the patients on wheelchairs are between the ages of 16 and 65. She does not understand why some of them have their medical bills covered by Medicare or Medicaid. What criteria make it possible for these patients to be covered?

_____

_____

_____

_____

6. A patient who just had his sixty-fifth birthday complains that Medicare is supposed to cover his insurance, but he says his first Social Security check showed a deduction for Medicare. What do you tell him?

_____

_____

_____

_____

_____

7. One of your patients is extremely concerned about the confidentiality of her medical records, especially after she learned that you transmit and store records electronically. She asks you how she can be assured that you will not "give too much information away."

_____

_____

_____

8. A patient at Walken and Thomisini has been out of work for six months because of a broken leg she sustained when she fell from a telephone pole after examining a line problem. Insurance from work has paid all her bills and provides her an income. Her husband, a farmer, caught his hand in a hay baler and cannot work, yet no insurance pays for him. She does not understand and asks you to explain.

_____

_____

_____

_____

9. An elderly patient tells you she never signs anything without thoroughly understanding it. One line of your patient information forms asks the patient to mark and sign a line called "Assignment of Benefits." She asks what this means.

_____

_____

_____

_____

10. You are training a medical assistant to become a CPT coder for the office. She asks you why the codes 99201 to 99499 are not designated to a particular specialty. What do you tell her?

_____

_____

_____

11. The billing task in your office is extremely demanding, one that requires the billing employees to work late several days a week. As office manager, you have been asked whether the audit trail function can be ignored for a few weeks while the staff catches up. What is your reply and why?

_____

_____

_____

_____

Simulation 14

Today is your fourteenth day of work at Marks and Graupera.

Supplies Needed

Five Health Insurance Claim Forms
One Workers' Compensation Insurance Form
To Do List
Work Summary

Action Options, Suggestions, and Conflicts

• Use your judgment in completing today's Action Papers.

Action Paper 14-1a

Marks and Graupera, P.C.

Note from Lydia

A couple of days ago, you completed the patient charge slips for the following patients:

Arash Bonaker
Angela Swazer
Sandra Hight
Cynthia Rambo
Margaret Stryker

Please prepare a health insurance claim form for each. Attach the patient charge slip to the bottom of the form. This eliminates the need to fill in every box.

PLEASE
DO NOT
STAPLE
IN THIS
AREA

APPROVED OMB-0938-0008

CARRIER

| | | | | | PICA | | **HEALTH INSURANCE CLAIM FORM** | PICA | |

1. MEDICARE	MEDICAID	CHAMPUS	CHAMPVA	GROUP HEALTH PLAN	FECA BLK LUNG	OTHER	1a. INSURED'S I.D. NUMBER	(FOR PROGRAM IN ITEM 1)
☐ (Medicare #)	☐ (Medicaid #)	☐ (Sponsor's SSN)	☐ (VA File #)	☐ (SSN or ID)	☐ (SSN)	☐ (ID)		

2. PATIENT'S NAME (Last Name, First Name, Middle Initial)	3. PATIENT'S BIRTH DATE MM	DD	YY SEX M ☐ F ☐	4. INSURED'S NAME (Last Name, First Name, Middle Initial)

5. PATIENT'S ADDRESS (No., Street)

6. PATIENT RELATIONSHIP TO INSURED

Self ☐ Spouse ☐ Child ☐ Other ☐

7. INSURED'S ADDRESS (No., Street)

CITY | STATE

8. PATIENT STATUS

Single ☐ Married ☐ Other ☐

Employed ☐ Full-Time Student ☐ Part-Time Student ☐

CITY | STATE

ZIP CODE | TELEPHONE (Include Area Code)

ZIP CODE | TELEPHONE (INCLUDE AREA CODE)

9. OTHER INSURED'S NAME (Last Name, First Name, Middle Initial)

10. IS PATIENT'S CONDITION RELATED TO:

11. INSURED'S POLICY GROUP OR FECA NUMBER

a. OTHER INSURED'S POLICY OR GROUP NUMBER

a. EMPLOYMENT? (CURRENT OR PREVIOUS)
☐ YES ☐ NO

a. INSURED'S DATE OF BIRTH MM | DD | YY SEX M ☐ F ☐

b. OTHER INSURED'S DATE OF BIRTH MM | DD | YY SEX M ☐ F ☐

b. AUTO ACCIDENT? PLACE (State)
☐ YES ☐ NO

b. EMPLOYER'S NAME OR SCHOOL NAME

c. EMPLOYER'S NAME OR SCHOOL NAME

c. OTHER ACCIDENT?
☐ YES ☐ NO

c. INSURANCE PLAN NAME OR PROGRAM NAME

d. INSURANCE PLAN NAME OR PROGRAM NAME

10d. RESERVED FOR LOCAL USE

d. IS THERE ANOTHER HEALTH BENEFIT PLAN?
☐ YES ☐ NO **If yes,** return to and complete item 9 a-d.

READ BACK OF FORM BEFORE COMPLETING & SIGNING THIS FORM.

12. PATIENT'S OR AUTHORIZED PERSON'S SIGNATURE I authorize the release of any medical or other information necessary to process this claim. I also request payment of government benefits either to myself or to the party who accepts assignment below.

SIGNED _____ DATE _____

13. INSURED'S OR AUTHORIZED PERSON'S SIGNATURE I authorize payment of medical benefits to the undersigned physician or supplier for services described below.

SIGNED _____

PATIENT AND INSURED INFORMATION

14. DATE OF CURRENT: MM	DD	YY ◄ ILLNESS (First symptom) OR INJURY (Accident) OR PREGNANCY(LMP)	15. IF PATIENT HAS HAD SAME OR SIMILAR ILLNESS. GIVE FIRST DATE MM	DD	YY	16. DATES PATIENT UNABLE TO WORK IN CURRENT OCCUPATION MM	DD	YY FROM TO MM	DD	YY

17. NAME OF REFERRING PHYSICIAN OR OTHER SOURCE

17a. I.D. NUMBER OF REFERRING PHYSICIAN

18. HOSPITALIZATION DATES RELATED TO CURRENT SERVICES MM | DD | YY FROM TO MM | DD | YY

19. RESERVED FOR LOCAL USE

20. OUTSIDE LAB?
☐ YES ☐ NO $ CHARGES

21. DIAGNOSIS OR NATURE OF ILLNESS OR INJURY. (RELATE ITEMS 1,2,3 OR 4 TO ITEM 24E BY LINE)

1. L___.___   3. L___.___

2. L___.___   4. L___.___

22. MEDICAID RESUBMISSION CODE ORIGINAL REF. NO.

23. PRIOR AUTHORIZATION NUMBER

24. A DATE(S) OF SERVICE From To MM DD YY MM DD YY	B Place of Service	C Type of Service	D PROCEDURES, SERVICES, OR SUPPLIES (Explain Unusual Circumstances) CPT/HCPCS MODIFIER	E DIAGNOSIS CODE	F $ CHARGES	G DAYS OR UNITS	H EPSDT Family Plan	I EMG	J COB	K RESERVED FOR LOCAL USE
1										
2										
3										
4										
5										
6										

25. FEDERAL TAX I.D. NUMBER SSN ☐ EIN ☐	26. PATIENT'S ACCOUNT NO.	27. ACCEPT ASSIGNMENT? (For govt. claims, see back) ☐ YES ☐ NO	28. TOTAL CHARGE $	29. AMOUNT PAID $	30. BALANCE DUE $

31. SIGNATURE OF PHYSICIAN OR SUPPLIER INCLUDING DEGREES OR CREDENTIALS (I certify that the statements on the reverse apply to this bill and are made a part thereof.)

SIGNED _____ DATE _____

32. NAME AND ADDRESS OF FACILITY WHERE SERVICES WERE RENDERED (If other than home or office)

33. PHYSICIAN'S, SUPPLIER'S BILLING NAME, ADDRESS, ZIP CODE & PHONE #

PIN# _____ GRP# _____

PHYSICIAN OR SUPPLIER INFORMATION

(APPROVED BY AMA COUNCIL ON MEDICAL SERVICE 8/88) **PLEASE PRINT OR TYPE**

FORM CMS-1500 (U2) (12-90)
FORM OWCP-1500 FORM RRB-1500

Action Paper 14-1c

APPROVED OMB-0938-0008

HEALTH INSURANCE CLAIM FORM

PLEASE
DO NOT
STAPLE
IN THIS
AREA

| | PICA | | PICA | | |

| 1. MEDICARE | MEDICAID | CHAMPUS | CHAMPVA | GROUP HEALTH PLAN | FECA BLK LUNG | OTHER | 1a. INSURED'S I.D. NUMBER | (FOR PROGRAM IN ITEM 1) |

(Medicare #) (Medicaid #) (Sponsor's SSN) (VA File #) (SSN or ID) (SSN) (ID)

2. PATIENT'S NAME (Last Name, First Name, Middle Initial)

3. PATIENT'S BIRTH DATE   MM   DD   YY   SEX   M   F

4. INSURED'S NAME (Last Name, First Name, Middle Initial)

5. PATIENT'S ADDRESS (No., Street)

6. PATIENT RELATIONSHIP TO INSURED   Self   Spouse   Child   Other

7. INSURED'S ADDRESS (No., Street)

CITY   STATE

8. PATIENT STATUS   Single   Married   Other

CITY   STATE

ZIP CODE   TELEPHONE (Include Area Code)

Employed   Full-Time Student   Part-Time Student

ZIP CODE   TELEPHONE (INCLUDE AREA CODE)

9. OTHER INSURED'S NAME (Last Name, First Name, Middle Initial)

10. IS PATIENT'S CONDITION RELATED TO:

11. INSURED'S POLICY GROUP OR FECA NUMBER

a. OTHER INSURED'S POLICY OR GROUP NUMBER

a. EMPLOYMENT? (CURRENT OR PREVIOUS)   YES   NO

a. INSURED'S DATE OF BIRTH   MM   DD   YY   SEX   M   F

b. OTHER INSURED'S DATE OF BIRTH   MM   DD   YY   SEX   M   F

b. AUTO ACCIDENT?   PLACE (State)   YES   NO

b. EMPLOYER'S NAME OR SCHOOL NAME

c. EMPLOYER'S NAME OR SCHOOL NAME

c. OTHER ACCIDENT?   YES   NO

c. INSURANCE PLAN NAME OR PROGRAM NAME

d. INSURANCE PLAN NAME OR PROGRAM NAME

10d. RESERVED FOR LOCAL USE

d. IS THERE ANOTHER HEALTH BENEFIT PLAN?   YES   NO   If yes, return to and complete item 9 a-d.

READ BACK OF FORM BEFORE COMPLETING & SIGNING THIS FORM.

12. PATIENT'S OR AUTHORIZED PERSON'S SIGNATURE I authorize the release of any medical or other information necessary to process this claim. I also request payment of government benefits either to myself or to the party who accepts assignment below.

SIGNED _____   DATE _____

13. INSURED'S OR AUTHORIZED PERSON'S SIGNATURE I authorize payment of medical benefits to the undersigned physician or supplier for services described below.

SIGNED _____

14. DATE OF CURRENT: MM   DD   YY   ILLNESS (First symptom) OR INJURY (Accident) OR PREGNANCY(LMP)

15. IF PATIENT HAS HAD SAME OR SIMILAR ILLNESS. GIVE FIRST DATE   MM   DD   YY

16. DATES PATIENT UNABLE TO WORK IN CURRENT OCCUPATION   MM   DD   YY   TO   MM   DD   YY   FROM

17. NAME OF REFERRING PHYSICIAN OR OTHER SOURCE

17a. I.D. NUMBER OF REFERRING PHYSICIAN

18. HOSPITALIZATION DATES RELATED TO CURRENT SERVICES   MM   DD   YY   TO   MM   DD   YY   FROM

19. RESERVED FOR LOCAL USE

20. OUTSIDE LAB?   YES   NO $ CHARGES

21. DIAGNOSIS OR NATURE OF ILLNESS OR INJURY. (RELATE ITEMS 1,2,3 OR 4 TO ITEM 24E BY LINE)

1. _____ . _____   3. _____ . _____

2. _____ . _____   4. _____ . _____

22. MEDICAID RESUBMISSION CODE   ORIGINAL REF. NO.

23. PRIOR AUTHORIZATION NUMBER

24. A DATE(S) OF SERVICE From To MM DD YY MM DD YY	B Place of Service	C Type of Service	D PROCEDURES, SERVICES, OR SUPPLIES (Explain Unusual Circumstances) CPT/HCPCS	MODIFIER	E DIAGNOSIS CODE	F $ CHARGES	G DAYS OR UNITS	H EPSDT Family Plan	I EMG	J COB	K RESERVED FOR LOCAL USE
1											
2											
3											
4											
5											
6											

25. FEDERAL TAX I.D. NUMBER   SSN   EIN

26. PATIENT'S ACCOUNT NO.

27. ACCEPT ASSIGNMENT? (For govt. claims, see back)   YES   NO

28. TOTAL CHARGE $

29. AMOUNT PAID $

30. BALANCE DUE $

31. SIGNATURE OF PHYSICIAN OR SUPPLIER INCLUDING DEGREES OR CREDENTIALS (I certify that the statements on the reverse apply to this bill and are made a part thereof.)

SIGNED _____   DATE _____

32. NAME AND ADDRESS OF FACILITY WHERE SERVICES WERE RENDERED (If other than home or office)

33. PHYSICIAN'S, SUPPLIER'S BILLING NAME, ADDRESS, ZIP CODE & PHONE #

PIN#   GRP#

(APPROVED BY AMA COUNCIL ON MEDICAL SERVICE 8/88)   **PLEASE PRINT OR TYPE**

FORM CMS-1500 (U2) (12-90)
FORM OWCP-1500   FORM RRB-1500

CARRIER — PATIENT AND INSURED INFORMATION — PHYSICIAN OR SUPPLIER INFORMATION

Name: _____   Date: _____

Action Paper 14-1d

APPROVED OMB-0938-0008

CARRIER

| | PICA | | **HEALTH INSURANCE CLAIM FORM** | | PICA | |

1. MEDICARE MEDICAID CHAMPUS CHAMPVA GROUP HEALTH PLAN FECA BLK LUNG OTHER	1a. INSURED'S I.D. NUMBER (FOR PROGRAM IN ITEM 1)
(Medicare #) (Medicaid #) (Sponsor's SSN) (VA File #) (SSN or ID) (SSN) (ID)	

2. PATIENT'S NAME (Last Name, First Name, Middle Initial)	3. PATIENT'S BIRTH DATE MM DD YY SEX M F	4. INSURED'S NAME (Last Name, First Name, Middle Initial)
5. PATIENT'S ADDRESS (No., Street)	6. PATIENT RELATIONSHIP TO INSURED Self Spouse Child Other	7. INSURED'S ADDRESS (No., Street)
CITY STATE	8. PATIENT STATUS Single Married Other	CITY STATE
ZIP CODE TELEPHONE (Include Area Code)	Employed Full-Time Student Part-Time Student	ZIP CODE TELEPHONE (INCLUDE AREA CODE)
9. OTHER INSURED'S NAME (Last Name, First Name, Middle Initial)	10. IS PATIENT'S CONDITION RELATED TO:	11. INSURED'S POLICY GROUP OR FECA NUMBER
a. OTHER INSURED'S POLICY OR GROUP NUMBER	a. EMPLOYMENT? (CURRENT OR PREVIOUS) YES NO	a. INSURED'S DATE OF BIRTH MM DD YY SEX M F
b. OTHER INSURED'S DATE OF BIRTH MM DD YY SEX M F	b. AUTO ACCIDENT? PLACE (State) YES NO	b. EMPLOYER'S NAME OR SCHOOL NAME
c. EMPLOYER'S NAME OR SCHOOL NAME	c. OTHER ACCIDENT? YES NO	c. INSURANCE PLAN NAME OR PROGRAM NAME
d. INSURANCE PLAN NAME OR PROGRAM NAME	10d. RESERVED FOR LOCAL USE	d. IS THERE ANOTHER HEALTH BENEFIT PLAN? YES NO If yes, return to and complete item 9 a-d.

READ BACK OF FORM BEFORE COMPLETING & SIGNING THIS FORM.

12. PATIENT'S OR AUTHORIZED PERSON'S SIGNATURE I authorize the release of any medical or other information necessary to process this claim. I also request payment of government benefits either to myself or to the party who accepts assignment below. SIGNED _____ DATE _____	13. INSURED'S OR AUTHORIZED PERSON'S SIGNATURE I authorize payment of medical benefits to the undersigned physician or supplier for services described below. SIGNED _____

PATIENT AND INSURED INFORMATION

14. DATE OF CURRENT: MM DD YY ILLNESS (First symptom) OR INJURY (Accident) OR PREGNANCY(LMP)	15. IF PATIENT HAS HAD SAME OR SIMILAR ILLNESS. GIVE FIRST DATE MM DD YY	16. DATES PATIENT UNABLE TO WORK IN CURRENT OCCUPATION MM DD YY FROM TO MM DD YY
17. NAME OF REFERRING PHYSICIAN OR OTHER SOURCE	17a. I.D. NUMBER OF REFERRING PHYSICIAN	18. HOSPITALIZATION DATES RELATED TO CURRENT SERVICES MM DD YY FROM TO MM DD YY
19. RESERVED FOR LOCAL USE		20. OUTSIDE LAB? YES NO $ CHARGES
21. DIAGNOSIS OR NATURE OF ILLNESS OR INJURY. (RELATE ITEMS 1,2,3 OR 4 TO ITEM 24E BY LINE) 1. ____ . ____ 3. ____ . ____ 2. ____ . ____ 4. ____ . ____		22. MEDICAID RESUBMISSION CODE ORIGINAL REF. NO. 23. PRIOR AUTHORIZATION NUMBER

24. A. DATE(S) OF SERVICE					B. Place of Service	C. Type of Service	D. PROCEDURES, SERVICES, OR SUPPLIES (Explain Unusual Circumstances) CPT/HCPCS	MODIFIER	E. DIAGNOSIS CODE	F. $ CHARGES	G. DAYS OR UNITS	H. EPSDT Family Plan	I. EMG	J. COB	K. RESERVED FOR LOCAL USE
From MM	DD	YY	To MM	DD	YY											
1															
2															
3															
4															
5															
6															

PHYSICIAN OR SUPPLIER INFORMATION

25. FEDERAL TAX I.D. NUMBER SSN EIN	26. PATIENT'S ACCOUNT NO.	27. ACCEPT ASSIGNMENT? (For govt. claims, see back) YES NO	28. TOTAL CHARGE $	29. AMOUNT PAID $	30. BALANCE DUE $
31. SIGNATURE OF PHYSICIAN OR SUPPLIER INCLUDING DEGREES OR CREDENTIALS (I certify that the statements on the reverse apply to this bill and are made a part thereof.) SIGNED _____ DATE _____	32. NAME AND ADDRESS OF FACILITY WHERE SERVICES WERE RENDERED (If other than home or office)		33. PHYSICIAN'S, SUPPLIER'S BILLING NAME, ADDRESS, ZIP CODE & PHONE # PIN# GRP#		

(APPROVED BY AMA COUNCIL ON MEDICAL SERVICE 8/88)   **PLEASE PRINT OR TYPE**   FORM CMS-1500 (U2) (12-90)   FORM OWCP-1500   FORM RRB-1500

Action Paper 14-1e

APPROVED OMB-0938-0008

CARRIER

[ ] PICA

HEALTH INSURANCE CLAIM FORM

PICA [ ][ ]

1. MEDICARE	MEDICAID	CHAMPUS	CHAMPVA	GROUP HEALTH PLAN	FECA BLK LUNG	OTHER	1a. INSURED'S I.D. NUMBER (FOR PROGRAM IN ITEM 1)
(Medicare #)	(Medicaid #)	(Sponsor's SSN)	(VA File #)	(SSN or ID)	(SSN)	(ID)	

2. PATIENT'S NAME (Last Name, First Name, Middle Initial)

3. PATIENT'S BIRTH DATE MM DD YY   SEX M [ ] F [ ]

4. INSURED'S NAME (Last Name, First Name, Middle Initial)

5. PATIENT'S ADDRESS (No., Street)

6. PATIENT RELATIONSHIP TO INSURED
Self [ ] Spouse [ ] Child [ ] Other [ ]

7. INSURED'S ADDRESS (No., Street)

CITY   STATE

8. PATIENT STATUS
Single [ ] Married [ ] Other [ ]

Employed [ ] Full-Time Student [ ] Part-Time Student [ ]

CITY   STATE

ZIP CODE   TELEPHONE (Include Area Code)

ZIP CODE   TELEPHONE (INCLUDE AREA CODE)

9. OTHER INSURED'S NAME (Last Name, First Name, Middle Initial)

10. IS PATIENT'S CONDITION RELATED TO:

11. INSURED'S POLICY GROUP OR FECA NUMBER

a. OTHER INSURED'S POLICY OR GROUP NUMBER

a. EMPLOYMENT? (CURRENT OR PREVIOUS)
YES [ ] NO [ ]

a. INSURED'S DATE OF BIRTH MM DD YY   SEX M [ ] F [ ]

b. OTHER INSURED'S DATE OF BIRTH MM DD YY SEX M [ ] F [ ]

b. AUTO ACCIDENT?   PLACE (State)
YES [ ] NO [ ]

b. EMPLOYER'S NAME OR SCHOOL NAME

c. EMPLOYER'S NAME OR SCHOOL NAME

c. OTHER ACCIDENT?
YES [ ] NO [ ]

c. INSURANCE PLAN NAME OR PROGRAM NAME

d. INSURANCE PLAN NAME OR PROGRAM NAME

10d. RESERVED FOR LOCAL USE

d. IS THERE ANOTHER HEALTH BENEFIT PLAN?
YES [ ] NO [ ] If yes, return to and complete item 9 a-d.

READ BACK OF FORM BEFORE COMPLETING & SIGNING THIS FORM.

12. PATIENT'S OR AUTHORIZED PERSON'S SIGNATURE I authorize the release of any medical or other information necessary to process this claim. I also request payment of government benefits either to myself or to the party who accepts assignment below.

SIGNED _____ DATE _____

13. INSURED'S OR AUTHORIZED PERSON'S SIGNATURE I authorize payment of medical benefits to the undersigned physician or supplier for services described below.

SIGNED _____

14. DATE OF CURRENT: ILLNESS (First symptom) OR INJURY (Accident) OR PREGNANCY(LMP) MM DD YY

15. IF PATIENT HAS HAD SAME OR SIMILAR ILLNESS. GIVE FIRST DATE MM DD YY

16. DATES PATIENT UNABLE TO WORK IN CURRENT OCCUPATION
FROM MM DD YY TO MM DD YY

17. NAME OF REFERRING PHYSICIAN OR OTHER SOURCE

17a. I.D. NUMBER OF REFERRING PHYSICIAN

18. HOSPITALIZATION DATES RELATED TO CURRENT SERVICES
FROM MM DD YY TO MM DD YY

19. RESERVED FOR LOCAL USE

20. OUTSIDE LAB?
YES [ ] NO [ ] $ CHARGES

21. DIAGNOSIS OR NATURE OF ILLNESS OR INJURY. (RELATE ITEMS 1,2,3 OR 4 TO ITEM 24E BY LINE)

1. L___.___   3. L___.___
2. L___.___   4. L___.___

22. MEDICAID RESUBMISSION CODE   ORIGINAL REF. NO.

23. PRIOR AUTHORIZATION NUMBER

24. A		B	C	D		E	F	G	H	I	J	K
DATE(S) OF SERVICE From To		Place of Service	Type of Service	PROCEDURES, SERVICES, OR SUPPLIES (Explain Unusual Circumstances) CPT/HCPCS MODIFIER		DIAGNOSIS CODE	$ CHARGES	DAYS OR UNITS	EPSDT Family Plan	EMG	COB	RESERVED FOR LOCAL USE
MM DD YY	MM DD YY											
1												
2												
3												
4												
5												
6												

25. FEDERAL TAX I.D. NUMBER   SSN [ ] EIN [ ]

26. PATIENT'S ACCOUNT NO.

27. ACCEPT ASSIGNMENT? (For govt. claims, see back)
YES [ ] NO [ ]

28. TOTAL CHARGE $

29. AMOUNT PAID $

30. BALANCE DUE $

31. SIGNATURE OF PHYSICIAN OR SUPPLIER INCLUDING DEGREES OR CREDENTIALS (I certify that the statements on the reverse apply to this bill and are made a part thereof.)

SIGNED _____ DATE _____

32. NAME AND ADDRESS OF FACILITY WHERE SERVICES WERE RENDERED (If other than home or office)

33. PHYSICIAN'S, SUPPLIER'S BILLING NAME, ADDRESS, ZIP CODE & PHONE #

PIN# _____ GRP# _____

(APPROVED BY AMA COUNCIL ON MEDICAL SERVICE 8/88)   **PLEASE PRINT OR TYPE**   FORM CMS-1500 (U2) (12-90) FORM OWCP-1500   FORM RRB-1500

PLEASE
DO NOT
STAPLE
IN THIS
AREA

APPROVED OMB-0938-0008

CARRIER

| | PICA | | | **HEALTH INSURANCE CLAIM FORM** | | PICA | |

HEALTH INSURANCE CLAIM FORM

1. MEDICARE	MEDICAID	CHAMPUS	CHAMPVA	GROUP HEALTH PLAN	FECA BLK LUNG	OTHER	1a. INSURED'S I.D. NUMBER	(FOR PROGRAM IN ITEM 1)
(Medicare #)	(Medicaid #)	(Sponsor's SSN)	(VA File #)	(SSN or ID)	(SSN)	(ID)		

2. PATIENT'S NAME (Last Name, First Name, Middle Initial)

3. PATIENT'S BIRTH DATE
MM   DD   YY   SEX
M ☐   F ☐

4. INSURED'S NAME (Last Name, First Name, Middle Initial)

5. PATIENT'S ADDRESS (No., Street)

6. PATIENT RELATIONSHIP TO INSURED
Self ☐   Spouse ☐   Child ☐   Other ☐

7. INSURED'S ADDRESS (No., Street)

CITY   STATE

8. PATIENT STATUS
Single ☐   Married ☐   Other ☐
Employed ☐   Full-Time Student ☐   Part-Time Student ☐

CITY   STATE

ZIP CODE   TELEPHONE (Include Area Code)

ZIP CODE   TELEPHONE (INCLUDE AREA CODE)

9. OTHER INSURED'S NAME (Last Name, First Name, Middle Initial)

10. IS PATIENT'S CONDITION RELATED TO:

11. INSURED'S POLICY GROUP OR FECA NUMBER

a. OTHER INSURED'S POLICY OR GROUP NUMBER

a. EMPLOYMENT? (CURRENT OR PREVIOUS)
☐ YES   ☐ NO

a. INSURED'S DATE OF BIRTH
MM   DD   YY   SEX
M ☐   F ☐

b. OTHER INSURED'S DATE OF BIRTH
MM   DD   YY   SEX
M ☐   F ☐

b. AUTO ACCIDENT?   PLACE (State)
☐ YES   ☐ NO

b. EMPLOYER'S NAME OR SCHOOL NAME

c. EMPLOYER'S NAME OR SCHOOL NAME

c. OTHER ACCIDENT?
☐ YES   ☐ NO

c. INSURANCE PLAN NAME OR PROGRAM NAME

d. INSURANCE PLAN NAME OR PROGRAM NAME

10d. RESERVED FOR LOCAL USE

d. IS THERE ANOTHER HEALTH BENEFIT PLAN?
☐ YES   ☐ NO   *If yes*, return to and complete item 9 a-d.

READ BACK OF FORM BEFORE COMPLETING & SIGNING THIS FORM.
12. PATIENT'S OR AUTHORIZED PERSON'S SIGNATURE I authorize the release of any medical or other information necessary to process this claim. I also request payment of government benefits either to myself or to the party who accepts assignment below.

SIGNED _____   DATE _____

13. INSURED'S OR AUTHORIZED PERSON'S SIGNATURE I authorize payment of medical benefits to the undersigned physician or supplier for services described below.

SIGNED _____

PATIENT AND INSURED INFORMATION

14. DATE OF CURRENT:
MM   DD   YY
◄ ILLNESS (First symptom) OR INJURY (Accident) OR PREGNANCY(LMP)

15. IF PATIENT HAS HAD SAME OR SIMILAR ILLNESS.
GIVE FIRST DATE   MM   DD   YY

16. DATES PATIENT UNABLE TO WORK IN CURRENT OCCUPATION
MM   DD   YY   MM   DD   YY
FROM   TO

17. NAME OF REFERRING PHYSICIAN OR OTHER SOURCE

17a. I.D. NUMBER OF REFERRING PHYSICIAN

18. HOSPITALIZATION DATES RELATED TO CURRENT SERVICES
MM   DD   YY   MM   DD   YY
FROM   TO

19. RESERVED FOR LOCAL USE

20. OUTSIDE LAB? $ CHARGES
☐ YES   ☐ NO

21. DIAGNOSIS OR NATURE OF ILLNESS OR INJURY. (RELATE ITEMS 1,2,3 OR 4 TO ITEM 24E BY LINE)
1. └___ . ___   3. └___ . ___
2. └___ . ___   4. └___ . ___

22. MEDICAID RESUBMISSION CODE   ORIGINAL REF. NO.

23. PRIOR AUTHORIZATION NUMBER

24. A DATE(S) OF SERVICE					B	C	D PROCEDURES, SERVICES, OR SUPPLIES		E	F	G	H	I	J	K
From MM DD YY			To MM DD YY		Place of Service	Type of Service	(Explain Unusual Circumstances) CPT/HCPCS MODIFIER		DIAGNOSIS CODE	$ CHARGES	DAYS OR UNITS	EPSDT Family Plan	EMG	COB	RESERVED FOR LOCAL USE
1															
2															
3															
4															
5															
6															

PHYSICIAN OR SUPPLIER INFORMATION

25. FEDERAL TAX I.D. NUMBER   SSN ☐ EIN ☐

26. PATIENT'S ACCOUNT NO.

27. ACCEPT ASSIGNMENT? (For govt. claims, see back)
☐ YES   ☐ NO

28. TOTAL CHARGE $

29. AMOUNT PAID $

30. BALANCE DUE $

31. SIGNATURE OF PHYSICIAN OR SUPPLIER INCLUDING DEGREES OR CREDENTIALS
(I certify that the statements on the reverse apply to this bill and are made a part thereof.)

SIGNED _____   DATE _____

32. NAME AND ADDRESS OF FACILITY WHERE SERVICES WERE RENDERED (If other than home or office)

33. PHYSICIAN'S, SUPPLIER'S BILLING NAME, ADDRESS, ZIP CODE & PHONE #

PIN#   GRP#

(APPROVED BY AMA COUNCIL ON MEDICAL SERVICE 8/88)   ***PLEASE PRINT OR TYPE***

FORM CMS-1500 (U2) (12-90)
FORM OWCP-1500   FORM RRB-1500

Action Paper 14-2a

Note from Tarik

Joseph Ramos, one of our long-time patients, brought this Workers' Compensation Insurance Form in. Will you complete it for him, please. His address is 1702 Landon Drive, King of Paoli, PA 19301, and his Social Security number is 238-55-9382. He was born 3/24/68.

On January 16, 200– at 10:00 AM, Joseph cut his hand on a meat cutting machine at H&R Butcher Shop, 2201 Lancaster Highway, Devon, PA 19087. He has had severe bleeding, no broken bones, severe pain, and twelve sutures. Dr. Graupera prescribed Tylenol p.r.n. for pain. Joseph will be out of work for four days and can return full-time after that.

Name: _____ Date: _____

INSTRUCTIONS

1. Type answers to All questions and file original with the Workers' Compensation Commission within 72 hours after first treatment.
2. DO NOT FAIL to forward to the Workers' Compensation Commission PROGRESS REPORTS and FINAL REPORT upon discharge of patient.

	DO NOT WRITE IN THIS SPACE
WORKERS' COMPENSATION COMMISSION	**WCC CLAIM #**
	EMPLOYER'S REPORT Yes ☐ No ☐

This is First Report ☐   Progress Report ☐   Final Report ☐

EVERY QUESTION MUST BE ANSWERED AND FORM SIGNED

1. Name of Injured Person: _____ Soc. Sec. No. _____ D.O.B. _____ Sex M ☐ F ☐

2. Address: (No. and Street) _____ (City or Town) _____ (State) _____ (Zip Code)

3. Name and Address of Employer:

4. Date of Accident or Onset of Disease: _____ Hour: _____ A.M. ☐ P.M. ☐   5. Date Disability Began:

6. Patient's Description of Accident or Cause of Disease:

7. Medical description of Injury or Disease:

8. Will Injury result in:

(a) Permanent defect? Yes ☐ No ☐ If so, what?   (b) Disfigurement Yes ☐ No ☐

9. Causes, other than injury, contributing to patients condition:

10. Is patient suffering from any disease of the heart, lungs, brain, kidneys, blood, vascular system or any other disabling condition not due to this accident? Give particulars:

11. Is there any history or evidence present of previous accident or disease? Give particulars:

12. Has normal recovery been delayed for any reason? Give particulars:

13. Date of first treatment: _____ Who engaged your services?

14. Describe treatment given by you:

15. Were X-Rays taken: Yes ☐ No ☐   By whom? — (Name and Address) _____ Date

16. X-Ray Diagnosis:

17. Was patient treated by anyone else? Yes ☐ No ☐   By whom? — (Name and Address) _____ Date

18. Was patient hospitalized? Yes ☐ No ☐   Name and Address of Hospital _____ Date of Admission: _____ Date of Discharge:

19. Is further treatment needed? Yes ☐ No ☐   For how long? _____ 20. Patient was ☐ will be ☐ able to resume regular work on: _____ Patient was ☐ will be ☐ able to resume light work on:

21. If death ensued give date: _____ 22. Remarks: (Give any information of value not included above)

☞ 23. I am a qualified specialist in: _____ I am a duly licensed Physician in the State of: _____ I was graduated from Medical School (Name) _____ Year

Date of this report: _____ (Signed) _____

(This report must be signed PERSONALLY by Physician)

Address: _____ Phone: _____

Name: _____ Date: _____

To Do List

-
-
-
-
-
-
-
-
-
-
-
-
-
-
-
-

Name: _____

Date Started: _____ Date Completed: _____

Work Summary 14

Section 1

1. Record the numbers of the Action Papers marked "Rush." _____

2. Record the numbers of the Action Papers marked "ASAP." _____

3. Record the numbers of the Action Papers marked "Routine." _____

Section 2

4. Write the list of "To Do" items and the actions that were taken. When this section is complete, turn the Work Summary over to your instructor, who will evaluate your work and return it for your later use.

To Do   Action Taken

_____   _____

_____   _____

_____   _____

_____   _____

_____   _____

_____   _____

Section 3

5. You will receive two assessments for your work—one is based on time to complete the items and the other is based on quality of work. Your instructor will complete the Assessment portion of the Work Summary.

Points Received

_____

Time Required

20 points	90 minutes or less
15 points	100 minutes
10 points	110 minutes
5 points	120 minutes

Quality of Work   _____

Total Points _____

PART V   Becoming a Career Medical Assistant

CHAPTER 15
Seeking Employment

Chapter Outline

Finding and Keeping a Job
Researching Employment Opportunities
    School Employment Offices
    Newspaper Classified Advertisements
    Professional Organizations
    Acquaintances
    Employment Agencies
    Internet
    Yellow Pages
The Job Application Process
    The Resume
        Preparing a Resume
            Personal Information
            Career Objective
            Special Strengths
            Work Experience
            Education
            Honors and Awards
            Extracurricular Activities
            References
    Writing an Application Letter
        Procedures for Writing an Application Letter
    Completing an Application Form
    Providing Documentation
Interviewing for a Position
    Appearance
    Conduct
    Knowledge of the Employer
    Asking the Right Questions
        Illegal Questions
            Religion
            Marital Status
            Arrests
            Drug Testing
    Writing a Follow-Up Letter
Continuing the Education Process
    Re-certification
    Registered Medical Assistant
Office Management
    Personnel
    Fringe Benefits
    Patient Flow
    Facilities, Equipment, and Supplies Responsibilities
    Financial Matters
Chapter Activities
    Performance-Based Activities
    Expanding Your Thinking

Key Vocabulary Terms

Match each word or term with its correct meaning.

_____ 1. Application letter

_____ 2. Employment application

_____ 3. Resume

_____ 4. Credentialing

_____ 5. Employment agencies

_____ 6. Expectations

_____ 7. Networking

_____ 8. Recredentialing

a. standards of performance set by an individual or an employer

b. renewing a previously awarded recognition

c. a document that accompanies a resume based on the primary diagnosis

d. a standard form that identifies the places where an applicant has worked

e. verification that an individual has met certain industry standards

f. a formatted document listing an applicant's personal and employment information

g. companies that charge a fee to connect employers and job applicants

h. interacting with a circle of acquaintances

Chapter Review

1. Name several traits that a physician looks for in a medical assistant.

_____

_____

_____

_____

2. Name and describe several sources for finding employment.

_____

_____

_____

_____

3. Name and describe the contents of the major sections of a resume.

_____

_____

_____

_____

_____

4. Describe the components of a good application letter.

_____

_____

_____

_____

5. What can an applicant do to ensure an interview will go well?

_____

_____

_____

_____

6. What is the importance of certification and re-certification in obtaining a job?

_____

_____

_____

_____

7. Name several certifications that a medical assistant might obtain.

_____

_____

_____

_____

8. How do the duties of a medical office assistant and a medical office manager differ?

_____

_____

_____

_____

9. What fringe benefits might a medical office assistant expect from a job?

_____

_____

_____

_____

10. For which financial matters might a medical office manager be responsible?

_____

_____

_____

Critical Thinking Scenarios

1. Your friend Meredith is upset because Tabitha, another medical assistant, was selected for the job Meredith wanted at Norman and Lucas, P.C. She tells you that she knows Tabitha, a classmate whose grades were "only average." Meredith says, "She tries to make everyone like her. Sometimes she is so nice, it's annoying. My grades were a lot better than hers, and I can stand up for myself, even around testy patients." Why do you think Tabitha might have gotten the job instead of Meredith?

_____

_____

_____

_____

2. Even when no one is around, Jose will not share personal information about patients with you. In addition, Jose writes lengthy details in each patient's medical record for procedures he performs. When the office is not busy, instead of talking with you, he finds things to do. You have often wondered whether he does not trust you because he does not chat much. Patients like him because he seems to care about them and the staff likes him because he can be relied on. What are the characteristics Jose exhibits?

_____

_____

_____

_____

3. Sandy is having a hard time locating her first medical assistant job, so her dad, a pharmaceutical salesman, offers to mention her job search to some of the medical office managers he knows. Sandy says, "No, Dad, I want to find this job on my own. I would be embarrassed to have my parents help me." When her dad tells her he will introduce her to other people he knows in the medical field, she refuses. What important employment-seeking resource is Sandy ignoring? How should she handle the offer from her dad?

_____

_____

_____

_____

4. Ramon is in a hurry to get a job. He tells you that he is going to prepare one resume and "blanket the town" with it. What is wrong with this thinking?

_____

_____

_____

_____

5. Lorelei has spent weeks reading and responding to newspaper classified advertisements and searching for job opportunities on the Internet, yet she has not found a job that is suited to her background. Most of her classmates are already employed. Lorelei is shy and these methods of job searching are easiest for her. What recommendations would you make to her?

_____

_____

_____

_____

_____

6. Critique the following application letter, then explain to Margaritta how you think it should be changed.

To Whom It May Concern:

I am applying for the job as a medical assistant in your office because it seems like a job that would help me in my career. Although I just graduated from medical assisting school, I think I would do a good job. I am willing to learn.

I am including my resume as it gives all the information you will need about me. Please call me at 615-555-2345 for an interview, and I will give you my schedule.

Sincerely,
Margaritta Rubin

_____

_____

_____

_____

7. Before an important interview, Malik gets new cornrows for his hair. He carefully chooses which earring and bracelet to go with the slacks and coat he plans to wear. To be ready to complete the application, he tucks a pencil behind his ear. Although he does not know much about the employer, he identifies which bus route to take so he will be sure to arrive on time. When the office manager invites him in to her office, he relaxes in the comfortable chair and responds in a casual manner so she will recognize that he is confident. He does not ask any questions because he believes it is her responsibility to tell him anything he needs to know. How could Malik improve his chances for obtaining a job?

_____

_____

_____

_____

8. Although Dena is a very competent medical assistant, well liked by both the patients and staff, she seems stuck in her job. Another medical assistant, one who is equally qualified but who has been with the practice for a shorter period of time, has received a promotion to office manager. Dena complains to you that the only difference is that the other medical assistant has his certification. She says she just does not want to take the time to become certified and that her work should stand on its merits. What do you think of this philosophy?

_____

_____

_____

_____

9. As office manager, Suzanna is often so busy that she feels harassed. She is currently interviewing applicants for a medical assisting position, training a new medical assistant, working with the doctor on an employee benefit plan, and trying to obtain her certification. With so much to do, she has decided to forgo the usual background check of applicants for the medical assistant opening. Instead, she has decided on a medical assistant whose personality she likes and whose resume looks really good. What is wrong with this shortcut?

_____

_____

_____

_____

10. Almost as soon as Dr. Jordan opened her practice three years ago, it became very busy. Computers and other office equipment were ordered in a hurry and no maintenance agreements were purchased. The equipment breaks down fairly often because it is getting older. Currently, the staff tries to help each other with equipment problems and calls an expensive technician when they cannot resolve a technical problem themselves. What equipment recommendations would you make?

_____

_____

_____

_____

Simulation 15

Today is the last day of your training at Marks and Graupera. Now you are ready to tackle the work on your own.

Supplies Needed

Two sheets of blank paper
To Do List
Work Summary

Action Options, Suggestions, and Conflicts

• Make appropriate decisions to complete the Action Papers.

Action Paper 15-1

Note from Dr. Graupera

Though you've worked here only a few weeks, we're so busy that Dr. Marks and I have decided to hire another new medical assistant. We are pleased with the skills and characteristics you bring to the job. Will you please help us shortcut the interviewing process by listing the skills and characteristics you consider most important. We want to hire another person just like you!

Action Paper 15-2

Note from Lydia

Dr. Marks asked me what your plans are for becoming credentialed. Will you please respond on this note so I can get back to her with an answer? Thanks.

E-mail from Lydia

Hi, Dr. Graupera told me he wrote you a note about the new medical assistant we're hiring. Will you tell me what your expectations were when you interviewed with us so I can use this information to improve the interviewing process next time? Print a copy, please.

Thanks.

To Do List

-
-
-
-
-
-
-
-
-
-
-
-
-
-
-
-

Name: _____

Date Started: _____ Date Completed: _____

Work Summary 15

Section 1

1. Record the numbers of the Action Papers marked "Rush." _____

2. Record the numbers of the Action Papers marked "ASAP." _____

3. Record the numbers of the Action Papers marked "Routine." _____

Section 2

4. Write the list of "To Do" items and the actions that were taken. When this section is complete, turn the Work Summary over to your instructor, who will evaluate your work and return it for your later use.

To Do   Action Taken

_____   _____

_____   _____

_____   _____

_____   _____ ,

_____   _____

_____   _____

Section 3

5. You will receive two assessments for your work—one is based on time to complete the items and the other is based on quality of work. Your instructor will complete the Assessment portion of the Work Summary.

                                                            Points Received

Time Required   _____

          20 points   30 minutes or less
          15 points   35 minutes
          10 points   40 minutes
           5 points   45 minutes

Quality of Work (see Simulation 1 instructions)   _____

                                        Total Points _____